Blockchain for Secure Healthcare Using Internet of Medical Things (IoMT)

Sunil Gupta • Hitesh Kumar Sharma
Monit Kapoor

Blockchain for Secure Healthcare Using Internet of Medical Things (IoMT)

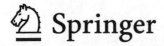

Sunil Gupta
University of Petroleum and Energy Studies
Dehradun, India

Hitesh Kumar Sharma
University of Petroleum and Energy Studies
Dehradun, India

Monit Kapoor
Chitkara University Institute of Engineering
and Technology
Punjab, India

ISBN 978-3-031-18898-5   ISBN 978-3-031-18896-1   (eBook)
https://doi.org/10.1007/978-3-031-18896-1

This Springer imprint is published by the registered company Springer Nature Switzerland AG
The registered company address is: Gewerbestrasse 11, 6330 Cham, Switzerland

Foreword

The Internet of Things is a combination of technologies and processes that are used to manage information retrieval from last-mile devices and create actionable insights after processing the data received from sensors. Internet of Medical Things (IoMT) is a special case of IoT that pertains to the collection, processing, and storage of data from patients so that they can be provided healthcare using sensor-based information. The main issue with healthcare-related data handling systems is the security and privacy data that belonging to patients and healthcare providers. Blockchain technology is a disruptive technology that ensures security, necessary privacy, and consistency in information sets all at the same time. The title of the book, i.e., "Blockchain for Secure Internet of Medical Things (IoMedT)" amply indicates the significance of blockchain technologies in the effective and secure management of healthcare-related tasks based on data acquisition made through medical sensors. This is a composite field involving computer science, mathematics, network management, and security issues.

The presence of communication networks in our lives is so pervasive and highly ubiquitous that it is next to impossible to ignore the presence of these networks in our daily lives. The interconnection of a large number of devices in our day-to-day life is demonstrating itself in multiple ways in various domains like banking, insurance, transportation, logistics, and healthcare. Analog watches have replaced themselves with smartwatches and fitness bands that most of us wear on our wrists and have found large-scale acceptance in our society in the last few years. Sensor-based systems are in use in healthcare with BPM monitors constantly providing a stream of data for the central team to observe and monitor. The various embedded gadgets are also used by medical professionals to keep track of patients under their care.

This book provides some valuable information on the integration of the domains of healthcare, the Internet of Things, and blockchain. The three technologies, if used wisely, can usher in a new era of pragmatic healthcare and ensure the security of data, which is critical to patients' well-being. The Internet of Medical Things is a domain of study that sits on top of the strength of IoT components-structural and functional and has medical sensors as the last mile device that transmits data about healthcare parameters. The IoMT can be a game changer for those geographies where there is a shortage of skilled healthcare professionals, as, through the usage of IOT-based communications, physicians sitting in different parts of the world can be alerted about health conditions and identify events around those conditions. Much has been achieved in terms of treating sensor data by driving it to cloud-based processing systems, and lots of actionable insights are created under the processing power of servers available in the cloud. The key always has been how secure data can be kept especially when it is about the health and well-being of individuals. This data, if it falls into malicious hands, can be used to wreak havoc of unimaginable proportions. Blockchain technologies by nature of it provide robust and trustworthy mechanisms to store, retrieve, and utilize data securely and efficiently. Blockchain has many use cases found in cryptocurrencies, risk assessment, land records management, and so on. Blockchain when put to use in managing healthcare parameters-related data of individuals can effectively allay fears of mishandling and illicit usage of data by parties who wish to exploit it for their wrongful needs. Blockchain has proven over time its effectiveness while providing security and privacy to data in other forms. This book promises to provide insights into how IoT and IoMT are related, and how these practices can benefit from blockchain technologies so that safety, security, and privacy issues are taken care of in a rightful manner.

Ever since the covid pandemic hit upon humanity, healthcare has become a highly discussed topic in all societies, rich or not so rich, around the globe. Technology has been our savior in our pursuit to nullify the effects of pandemics and immunize a large stratum of the human population around the world. This book has come at a relevant time and provides necessary technical insights into the domain of IoMT and the suitability of blockchain technology to supplement security challenges in IoMT.

The challenges on the Internet of Medical Things are both difficult and interesting. Researchers are working on them with lots of enthusiasm, a multitude of tenacity, and heartfelt dedication to developing new materials and methods of analysis. The aim is to provide cost-effective and secure solutions to keep up with the ever-changing threats to healthcare monitoring systems. In this present and forthcoming age of global hyper-connectivity and seamless interdependence, it is pertinent and obvious to provide IoMT scientists and researchers, security practitioners, professionals, and students with state-of-the-art knowledge on the contours of IoMT, healthcare systems, security, and blockchain. This book is a good step in that direction.

Vice Chancellor, University of Petroleum and Energy Studies   Sunil Rai,
Dehradun, India

Preface

The foundations of IoT and healthcare systems are covered in this book, including system designs, protocols, wearable technology, and interoperability. It looks at the main issues with artificial intelligence (AI) and smart computing in IoT-based applications with limited resources, as well as the costs, energy efficiency, and accessibility to high-quality services. The use of e-healthcare and telemedicine has facilitated remote patients' access to skilled medical professionals. Patients in distant communities can contact with medical specialists worldwide via mobile phones using telemedicine systems and eHealth services. These Internet platforms have aided society in receiving treatment from their place of abode during pandemic scenarios like COVID-19 without having to move their bodies. In order to enhance services and affect people's lives, technology is a critical component in the planning, designing, and development of intelligent systems. The book offers an interdisciplinary approach to the ideas of the Internet of Medical Things (IoMedT), IoT, and cloud computing adoption by bringing together cutting-edge research and views from researchers, academics, and practitioners around the world. The problem that humanity is facing is what is being presented to medicine. Real-time patient monitoring with adaptable wearable sensors and illness diagnosis using the greatest diagnostic tools are examples of innovations. This book's primary goal is to inform both novice and experienced users about telemedicine and smart healthcare. The use of smartphones and other electronic devices for disease diagnosis, bettering patient care, and enhancing quality of life is known as smart health technology. Healthcare organizations, providers, telemedicine agents, patients, and physicians can all have their present and future requirements met by technology. It is the populace's most recent and popular platform. The technology offers readily available resources to assist emergency response, extended use, increased communication, and improved impact. The distance between large medical facilities, like clinics, and providers, like general practitioners, is reduced because to this technology. The development of numerous technologies targeted at facilitating dependable, omnipresent communication between patients and healthcare professionals is required for end-to-end connectivity of clinical data. For the exchange of medical data between patients and healthcare professionals, MHealth and eHealth are essential elements of intelligent healthcare systems. In order to improve efficiency and patient care, smart healthcare decreases the time, cost, and risk associated with Internet of Things (IoT) healthcare implementations. Today, one of the largest obstacles to end-to-end delivery is protecting healthcare data. The Internet of Medical Things is a significant advancement that has given the healthcare sector an element of "intelligence," enabling service providers to recognize, monitor, and inform patients' clinical information to deliver medical services more quickly. The book is appropriate for a broad spectrum of academics who want to learn in-depth information about most recent IoMT-based solutions to healthcare issues.

Dehradun, India   Sunil Gupta
Punjab, India   Hitesh Kumar Sharma
                                                                               Monit Kapoor

Acknowledgement

As we draw close to finishing this project, our thoughts go to the day when we conceptualized this project and sent in a proposal to Springer Nature Group. Our joy knew no bounds when we received an email mentioning that our book proposal has been accepted. We place our sincere thanks to the Springer Nature group, Ms. Anna Harshvardhan and her team of superb individuals who have been extremely encouraging in our entire journey. Regarding any request we made to them, be it extension of a deadline or providing better insights to technical and logistic support for documentation, the Springer Nature team has been extremely forthcoming and highly mindful of our requirements.

We have been ably supported, advised, and motivated by our colleagues at Chitkara University and UPES, alike. Multiple rounds of discussions and ideation with colleagues have given the shape to the book as we all see it today. We are deeply indebted to university management both at UPES and Chitkara University for providing us excellent support from library through subscription of excellent journals, books, and related literature. The seamless availability has been a great motivation for us to spell out the chapters to the best to our capabilities.

We are deeply thankful to our better half and young children at home, for it was many a times their time as well that we bartered for working on this book. Family is the support system that helps one navigate through high and lows in lives, and there had been such times where a little procrastination did set in. But it was the right advice from our better halves in such moments that kept us going and we could finish this book project as per our agreed timelines.

We are deeply thankful to the Almighty, whose grace and benevolence has made us walk through this challenge with courage, grit, and self-esteem.

Contents

Abbreviations

AGAFL	Adaptive Genetic Algorithm with Fuzzy Logic
AI	Artificial Intelligence
API	Application Programming Interface
AWS	Amazon Web Service
BCA	Body Centric Applications
BYOD	Bring Your Own Device
CGM	Continuous Glucose Monitoring
CNN	Convolutional Neural Network
CNN-MDRP	Convolutional Neural Network-based Multimodal Disease Prediction
COVID	Coronavirus Disease
CPOE	Computerized Provider Order Entry
CSP	Cloud Service Providers
CT	Computed Tomography
DLT	Distributed Ledger Technology
ECG	Electrocardiogram
EDW	Enterprise Data Warehouses
EHR	Electronic Health Records
EHR/EMR	Electronic Health Records/Electronic Medical Records
EKG	Electrocardiogram
EMR	Electronic Medical Records
ETSI	European Telecommunications Standards Institute
FHIR	Fast Healthcare Interoperability Resources
GCP	Google Cloud Platform
GPS	Global Positioning System
GSM	Global System for Mobile Communication
HAPI	hospital-acquired pressure injury
HIT	Home Side Intervention
HITECH	Health Information Technology for Economic and Clinical Health Act
HITRUST	Health Information Trust Alliance

I2C	Inter-Integrated Circuit
IaaS	Infrastructure as a Service
IBM	International Business Machines
ICT	Information and Communications Technology
ICU	Intensive Care Unit
IEEE	Institute of Electrical and Electronics Engineers
IETF	Internet Engineering Task force
IIOT	Industrial Internet of Things
IoT	Internet of Things
IPFS	Interplanetary File Systems
IT	Information Technology
LTE	Long-Term Evolution
MAPE	Mean Absolute Percentage Error
ML	Machine Learning
MRI	Magnetic Resonance Imaging
NFV	Network Functions Virtualization
NLP	Natural Language Processing
OCA	Object Centric Applications
OPD	Out Patient Department
OTT	Over-The-Top
PAN	Personal Area Networks
PCB	Printed Circuit Board
PHI	Protected Health Information
PII	Personally Identifiable Information
RFID	Radio Frequency Identification
RIS	Regional Innovation System
RMSE	Root Mean Square Error
ROC	Registrars of Companies
RSA	Rivest-Shamir-Adleman
SC-UCSSO	SmartCard-Based User-Controlled Single Sign-On
SDN	Software-Defined Networking
SHA	Secure Hash Algorithm
SHS	Square Hollow Section
SMART	Substitutable Medical Applications, Reusable Technologies
SPI	Serial Peripheral Interface
UNICEF	United Nations International Children's Emergency Fund
UWB	Ultra-Wide Band
VPN	Virtual Private Network
WAN	Wide Area Network
WSN	Wireless Sensor Networks

Chapter 1
Introduction to Smart Healthcare and Telemedicine Systems

1.1 Introduction

"Health" is a self-evident word that describes the healthy ecosystem we are experiencing in our lives today. Smart healthcare is nothing more than using today's technology to make the existing healthcare ecosystem smart and intelligent. This can benefit patients, physicians, and the entire ecosystem, improving quality and patient care.

Telemedicine systems help reduce unnecessary congestion for individuals and government agencies. With the help of this type of telemedicine platform, rural patients can get medical advice from a variety of reputable hospitals and leading physicians available around the world. This approach improves the efficiency and availability of healthcare professionals and staff as needed. Traditional healthcare cannot meet the needs of everyone due to the significant population growth. Despite excellent infrastructure and cutting-edge technology, not everyone has access to or can afford medical care. Smart healthcare aims to assist consumers by teaching them about their health and increasing their awareness of it. Some emergencies can be self-managed by users of smart healthcare. The user experience and quality are being improved. Making the most of your available resources is made easier by smart healthcare. It enables remote patient monitoring and lowers the cost of user therapy. Additionally, it enables doctors to spread their services internationally. Effective smart healthcare systems ensure that inhabitants live healthy lives as the trend toward smart cities rises. Figure 1.1 shows the significant improvement of smart healthcare in comparison to traditional healthcare.

Healthcare is one of the most important sectors that require the integration of advanced technology. IoT-enabled sensors, electronic health record (EHR) storage, and advanced data analysis algorithms. Metaheuristic optimization techniques help traditional healthcare systems become intelligent healthcare systems. During the pandemic, recent developments in e-health and telemedicine systems have

© The Author(s), under exclusive license to Springer Nature Switzerland AG 2023
S. Gupta et al., *Blockchain for Secure Healthcare Using Internet of Medical Things (IoMT)*, https://doi.org/10.1007/978-3-031-18896-1_1

The traditional healthcare model	The Smart Healthcare Model
No better healthcare management is available.	Health authorities can get useful information regarding the efficiency of workers and equipment with the use of IoT devices.
It requires physical movement of the patient and doctor: Physical Monitoring	No Requirement for Physical Movement: Remote Monitoring
Medical records and prescriptions are stored in print or handwritten format with the hospital or patient.	Health records and prescriptions are stored digitally in cloud storage.
It involves more healthcare costs and time.	Reduce healthcare costs and time.
Real-time data with no storage	IoT Sensor is used for digital data and Cloud computing is used for storage
No way to track the drug administration and treatment response.	reducing medical errors and improving treatment management.
Physical face-to-face service is available	Hybrid care model that combines virtual services and face-to-face services
No use of Artificial Intelligence and Machine Learning	Use Artificial Intelligence and Machine Learning
No Advanced precision medicine	Advanced precision medicine
No advanced sensor is available to analyze and reduce the illness and acute condition	Intelligent sensors analyze health and reduce the incidence of illness and acute conditions

Fig. 1.1 Improvement of smart healthcare in comparison to traditional healthcare

demonstrated the importance and need for these healthcare advances. Smart health care and telemedicine are not the solutions to all health problems, but they can be used to treat many health problems without the physical movement of patients and doctors. Telemedicine systems help reduce unnecessary congestion in private and public hospitals. With the help of this type of telemedicine platform, rural patients can get health advice from a variety of reputable hospitals and talented doctors available around the world. This approach improves the efficiency and availability of specialists and medical staff as needed.

In today's digital age, smart healthcare has become one of the most important advances in healthcare. With advances in technology and scientific theory, traditional medicine based on biotechnology is gradually being digitized and beginning to provide information. With the increasing demand for quality health care and rising costs of care, comprehensive health care is seen as a technical solution for addressing global health problems. The Internet of Things (IoT), also known as the Internet of Healthcare Things (IoHT) or the Internet of Medical Things (IoMT), is anticipated to dramatically improve the efficiency and quality of care in the healthcare sector.

Due to developments in microelectronics, materials, and biosensor design, smart wearables and implantable medical devices, in particular, have drawn a lot of attention in recent years; nevertheless, these common, inexpensive sensor devices are now reactive. It might transform treatment into preventative medicine.

The IoMT system's main objective is to gather and transmit health data including EKG, weight, blood pressure, and blood sugar. Such data may be shared with physicians, participating healthcare providers, insurance providers, or authorized individuals who are external contractors, regardless of time, place, or device.

1.2   Smart Healthcare and Telemedical System

To connect healthcare-related individuals, resources, and institutions and to proactively satisfy the demands of the healthcare ecosystem. The smart healthcare system's many technologies are depicted in Fig. 1.2. A healthcare system controls and intelligently reacts to that. Patient-doctor contacts were only possible through visits, phone calls, and text messages before the Internet of Things. Doctors and facilities were unable to continuously assess the patient's condition and offer recommendations. Devices with the Internet of Things (IoT) capabilities enable remote healthcare monitoring, unleashing the potential for improved patient health and safety. Patient involvement and satisfaction grew as doctor-patient communication became simpler and more effective. Remote patient health monitoring can also shorten hospital stays and avoid readmissions [1].

1.2.1   Smart Healthcare Technology

With remote medicine, remote care, and health monitoring technology that connect patients and doctors in novel ways, healthcare smart technologies are revolutionizing how patients are treated. Here are some instances of how smart technology can be applied to the healthcare industry to enhance the patient experience, preventive care procedures, and global health [2].

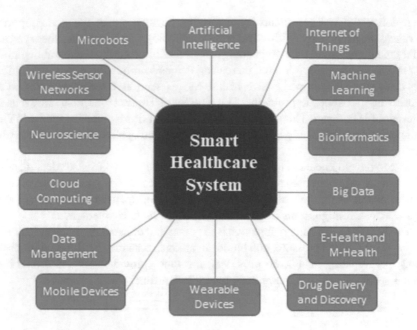

Fig. 1.2 Technology involved in smart healthcare

1.2.2   Remote Monitoring and Automated Healthcare System

A developing trend that transcends traditional health care and into popular culture is remote patient health monitoring. Smartwatches and fitness trackers have become commonplace for many people due to their capacity to monitor health markers including heart rate, blood oxygen levels, and arrhythmias. Healthcare practitioners are searching for medical equipment that helps patients by continuously monitoring their health and deciding on preventative treatments based on data patterns and expectations.

For instance, connected inhalers are smart medical device that helps patients monitor their consumption and reminds them when to take their medications to keep a healthy schedule [3].

1.2.3   Remote Care and Telehealth

We are all now familiar with telemedicine, which during the epidemic gained popularity among patients and healthcare professionals. Through video calls, conferencing technology enables professionals to virtually treat patients.

To assist clinicians and patients in tracking and wearing therapies, a portion of this virtual care makes use of medical portal technology to create a safe online health portal that you may use to store, gather, and access data from health records.

1.2.4 Emergency Response Solution for Connectivity

Connectivity has the power to save lives by greatly enhancing the effectiveness and response times of emergency care. To provide real-time reaction, the most recent intelligent healthcare technology enables quick data sharing between ambulances, physicians, first responders, accidents, and emergency departments.

Now made possible by new technologies that enable faster communications, video calls with doctors from within an ambulance, faster patient history acquisition, and easier hospitalization due to existing medical history and medical conditions. Upon arrival, doctors will have immediate access to patient data such as vital signs, blood pressure, heart rate, and temperature.

1.2.5 Smart Hospital Management

Intelligent hospital management is efficient by connecting digital systems for easy access to information such as bed occupancy, device usage, device status, number of materials and consumables, and other operational data. Helps improve effectiveness, improve the patient's experience, and assist doctors.

You can track this information and use it for decision-making to improve resource management, reduce waste, and avoid situations where you don't have what you need due to poor tracking or incorrect data collection.

1.3 Telemedical Healthcare

Telemedicine is intended to assist patients in accessing medical treatments from their homes. The concept of telemedicine has become very popular and useful during COVID-19. Figure 1.3 Illustrate Smart Healthcare with the Help of the Telemedicine Approach. According to the severity of the patient's symptoms, their age, and their location, advice, and medications are given based on this method's remote diagnosis of the patient's condition. Additionally, those that exhibit COVID-19 symptoms are excluded. In this paradigm, patients, telehealth service providers, and a central cloud-based telecare server are all present (or users). With any internet-enabled mobile device, patients can readily access healthcare services (phone, laptop, etc.). A doctor (healthcare provider), a cluster of doctors, a clinic, or a hospital are all examples of telehealth service providers, regardless of the location. The strategy includes actions made by both patients and clinicians.

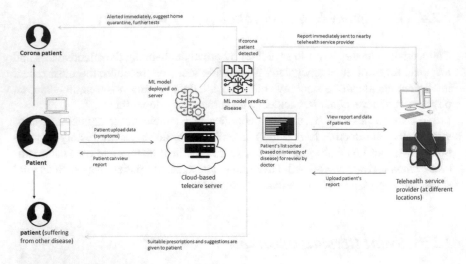

Fig. 1.3 Smart healthcare using telemedicine system

1.3.1 Registration Phase

Patient registration requires the patient to input their ID, password, and other credentials while using a mobile device. For security reasons, this data is first masked before being sent to the server. If the received identification with credentials does not already exist in the server database, the server examines the database, verifies the user using OTP, and registers the user.

Through a secure channel, telehealth service providers register, are verified and are then given an ID and password. Once enrolled, the provider of the telehealth service can log in using the specified ID and password to check on patients, access any shared data, and communicate with them.

1.3.2 Login Phase and Mutual Authentication

A timestamp is added as the patient inputs his ID and password, then sends them to the server. Users are authenticated by the server using their IDs, passwords, timestamps, and OTPs. A session key is generated and validated for future communication once the server successfully authenticates the patient, who then successfully authenticates both the server and the patient. To ensure secure transmission and access to the data, security procedures are used while sharing data. We do not employ biometrics for user convenience. Patients who live in remote areas or who are elderly might not have a fingerprint scanner.

The patient can examine his report and exchange the information with the telemedicine service provider after successfully logging in.

New patients must initially complete the form if they have any symptoms or a condition. A list of all COVID-19 symptoms is provided on this form. Patients might examine their symptoms to identify other, not-listed complaints. We will utilize this form in this instance because the patient may be unable to mention certain symptoms when speaking with the telecare server. The patient sends the Telecare server the form.

1.3.3 Telemedicine Server

A cloud-based Telecare server running the machine-learning model has been trained using historical patient data. Based on symptoms, this algorithm is taught to forecast sickness and its severity. This ML model may be configured to use continuous learning, allowing you to continuously learn from fresh datasets and keep track of evolving symptoms. The Telecare server forecasts the disease and its severity based on the information (symptoms) given by the patient.

Based on the expected illness and severity, make suggestions and prescribe medications when illnesses such as coughs and colds are easily cured. Patients are categorized according to their degree of illness, so patients do not have to look for a telemedicine service provider to see the right doctor. Patients with coronavirus fever symptoms are advised to stay in quarantine at home and take appropriate measures. The data will be sent to your local telecare service provider (entered during registration).

1.4 Intelligent Medical Care Using IoT

The Internet of Things will significantly affect how much money is spent on healthcare and how well patients do. There is little doubt that the Internet of Things (IoT) is disrupting the healthcare industry and altering how customers interact with technology and the delivery of healthcare solutions. IoT applications in healthcare are advantageous to patients, families, physicians, hospitals, and insurance providers. Wearable technology includes patient IoT fitness bands and wirelessly connected glucose meters, blood pressure cuffs, and heart rate monitors. The patient can get individualized care. These gadgets can be programmed to remind you of various things, including blood pressure changes, appointments, blood pressure checks, and calorie counting. By providing continuous health monitoring, especially for elderly patients, the internet of things has enhanced people's lives. The impact on people who live alone and their families is enormous. The alarm system tells concerned relatives and medical staff when a person's routine activities are interrupted or changed [4].

IoT for Doctors IoT-enabled wearables and other home security systems help doctors monitor patients' health more accurately. You can monitor a patient's adherence to a treatment regimen or whether they require emergency medical care. The Internet of Things (IoT) enables medical personnel to be more watchful and involved with their patients. Physicians can choose the best course of therapy for their patients and obtain the desired results with the help of the data gathered from IoT devices.

IoT for Hospitals IoT devices can be very helpful in hospitals in a variety of other ways outside only tracking patient health. Medical equipment like wheelchairs, defibrillators, nebulizers, oxygen pumps, and other surveillance devices are all employed in real-time placement thanks to sensor-tagged Internet of Things devices. Real-time analysis is also possible when deciding where to put healthcare workers. For hospital patients, infection transmission is a significant issue. The use of IoT-enabled hygiene monitoring equipment can help patients avoid contracting infections. IoT devices are also useful for environmental monitoring, such as regulating humidity and temperature and monitoring the refrigerator's temperature, as well as asset management, such as maintaining pharmacy inventory.

Health Insurers and IoT Health insurers can use smart devices connected to the IoT in a variety of ways. The information gathered by health monitoring devices can be used by insurance firms for underwriting and billing. They can find underwriting potential and detect fraud thanks to this data. IoT gadgets make the underwriting, pricing, billing, and risk assessment procedures transparent between insurers and clients. Customers can reasonably obtain insight into the underlying concepts behind each decision taken and the outcomes of operational processes thanks to the data-driven decisions gathered by the IoT in all operations. Customers might be encouraged by insurers to use and share health information produced by IoT devices. You may give your clients incentives for keeping track of their everyday activities, following treatment regimens and receiving preventive care by using IoT devices.

Numerous opportunities arise from the growth of IoT goods with a health focus. Additionally, the enormous amount of data that these linked devices produce has the potential to revolutionize healthcare [7]. The Internet of Things has a four-stage process architecture (see Fig. 1.4). Each of the four stages is related to the others so that information gathered or processed in one step can be useful in the next. The values incorporated into the process offer insight and a flexible business perspective.

Step 1: The first step is to utilize network devices, such as sensors, actuators, monitors, detectors, and camera systems, in the initial stage. These gadgets gather information.

Step 2: Analog data obtained from sensors and other devices is typically pooled and transformed into digital data to be processed further.

The data is preprocessed, standardized, and transferred to the data center or cloud once it has been digitized and aggregated.

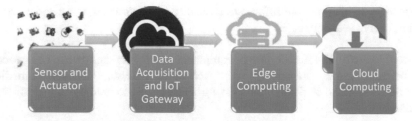

Fig. 1.4 Four-step architecture of IoT for smart healthcare

Step 3. The final data is managed and processed at the necessary level in step 4. The sophisticated analysis performed on this data offers useful commercial insights for sound decision-making.

By providing better care, improved patient outcomes, patient cost savings, better processes and workflows, increased performance, and improved patient experiences for healthcare providers, IoT is transforming healthcare. Increase. The Internet of Things in healthcare faces difficulties. Data security issues are brought up by the massive amounts of data that IoT-enabled linked devices collect, particularly sensitive data. Adequate security measures must be put in place [5, 6]. The Internet of Things is investigating new elements of patient care through real-time health monitoring and access to patient health data. Healthcare personnel can use this data to increase patient satisfaction and health, increase income prospects, and enhance operational efficiency. The ability to use this digital power effectively is becoming a more important differentiation in the linked world.

1.5 Smart Healthcare: Challenges and Threats

Medical information is extremely private and sensitive. The system's users' and doctors' personal information could be accessed and altered by an attacker. You must choose an eight-digit alphanumeric password with unusual characters to protect yourself from such attacks. OTP is required to improve user and system information security [8]. Data breaches and unprecedented monitoring are major concerns. Data must be sent securely encrypted. Use of the HTTPS protocol is required. Users must not divulge their personal information and authentication codes to third parties. They are required to keep their information on them. Without OTP, one cannot authenticate even if they have the user's credentials. Even while the IoT has a lot to offer the healthcare industry, there are still substantial obstacles that must be overcome before it can be widely adopted. The following are the dangers and drawbacks of employing linked devices in healthcare:

Security and Privacy Users are deterred from using IoT technology for medical purposes by serious security and privacy issues since healthcare monitoring technologies can be compromised or hacked. The advantages of the IoT can be seriously harmed by leaking private information about a patient's location or health, or by manipulating sensor data [9].

Risk of Failure The functioning of equipment attached to sensors can be impacted by hardware issues, breakdowns, and even power outages, endangering medical practice. It can also be riskier than missing health checks to ignore planned software updates.

Integration: Multiple Protocols and Different Devices Devices from various manufacturers could not function properly together due to a lack of consensus on IoT protocols and standards. The IoT's potential effectiveness is constrained by the absence of standardization, which prevents full integration. As a result, manufacturers may develop their ecosystem of Internet of Things (IoT) devices that are incompatible with the products and applications of other manufacturers. There isn't a synchronization technique that can be used in this case for data aggregation. The process is slowed down by this irregularity, which also limits the Healthcare IoT's potential to scale.

Cost Although the IoT promises to eventually save medical expenses, it will be exceedingly expensive to install in hospitals and train employees [10].

Overload of Data and Accuracy It is challenging to aggregate data for crucial insights and analysis because of the various data types and communication methods. The IoT performs proper data processing and large data collection. The data should be divided into manageable portions with accurate precision and without overloading for better results. Additionally, long-term decision-making in the hospitality sector may be hampered by data overload [11].

1.6   Conclusion

Smart health or telemedicine systems are not the solution to all health-related problems but can be used to solve many health problems without the physical movement of the patient or doctor. It helps reduce unnecessary amounts in private and public hospitals. With the help of this type of telemedicine platform, rural patients can receive medical advice from various reputable hospitals and leading doctors around the world.

   This approach improves the efficiency and availability of healthcare professionals and on-demand staff. The need for these types of systems also requires equal quality and security. Since these systems handle public health directly, they also require a strong and efficient authentication mechanism. This chapter provides the knowledge that patients can easily access medical services without having to physically attend the hospital. This approach is also suitable for older patients. Patients simply log in through the portal and send their symptoms to a cloud-based server.

Patients do not have to look for a doctor or visit a hospital. After receiving patient data, the Telecare server takes over the tasks of predicting illness, prescribing, filtering patient information, and sending data to telemedicine service providers using the appropriate ML model.

References

1. Sageena G, Sharma M, Kapur A. Evolution of Smart Healthcare: Telemedicine During COVID-19 Pandemic. J. Inst. Eng. India Ser. B. 2021;102(6):1319–24. doi: https://doi.org/10.1007/s40031-021-00568-8. Epub 2021 Apr 3. PMCID: PMC8019338.
2. Vyas, S., Bhargava, D. Smart Health: An Introduction. In: Smart Health Systems. Springer, Singapore. 2021, doi:https://doi.org/10.1007/978-981-16-4201-2_1
3. J. Anu Shilvya, S. Thomas George, M. S. P. Subathra, P. Manimegalai, Mazin Abed Mohammed, Mustafa Musa Jaber, Afsaneh Kazemzadeh, Mohammed Nasser Al-Andoli, "Home Based Monitoring for Smart Health-Care Systems: A Survey", Wireless Communications and Mobile Computing, vol. 2022, Article ID 1829876, 10 pages, 2022. doi:10.1155/2022/1829876
4. S. M. Nagarajan, G. G. Deverajan, K. Kumaran, M. Thirunavukkarasan, M. D. Alshehri and S. Alkhalaf, "Secure Data Transmission in Internet of Medical Things using RES-256 Algorithm," in IEEE Transactions on Industrial Informatics, doi: https://doi.org/10.1109/TII.2021.3126119.
5. Ghubaish, T. Salman, M. Zolanvari, D. Unal, A. Al Ali and R. Jain, "Recent Advances in the Internet-of-Medical-Things (IoMT) Systems Security," in IEEE Internet of Things Journal, vol. 8, no. 11, pp. 8707–8718, 1 June 1, 2021, doi: https://doi.org/10.1109/JIOT.2020.3045653.
6. M. Mushtaq, M. A. Shah and A. Ghafoor, "The Internet Of Medical Things (Iomt): Security Threats And Issues Affecting Digital Economy," Competitive Advantage in the Digital Economy (CADE 2021), 2021, pp. 137–142, doi: https://doi.org/10.1049/icp.2021.2420.
7. S. A. Parah et al., "Efficient Security and Authentication for Edge-Based Internet of Medical Things," in IEEE Internet of Things Journal, vol. 8, no. 21, pp. 15652–15662, 1 Nov. 1, 2021, doi: https://doi.org/10.1109/JIOT.2020.3038009.
8. M. Kumar and S. Chand, "A Secure and Efficient Cloud-Centric Internet-of-Medical-Things-Enabled Smart Healthcare System With Public Verifiability," in IEEE Internet of Things Journal, vol. 7, no. 10, pp. 10650–10659, Oct. 2020, doi: https://doi.org/10.1109/JIOT.2020.3006523.
9. R. Nidhya; Manish Kumar; R. Maheswar; D. Pavithra, "Security and Privacy Issues in Smart Healthcare System Using Internet of Things," in IoT-enabled Smart Healthcare Systems, Services and Applications, Wiley, 2022, pp. 63–85, doi: https://doi.org/10.1002/9781119816829.ch4.
10. Chen B, Baur A, Stepniak M, Wang J (2019) Finding the future of care provision: the role of smart hospitals. McKinsey & Company. https://www.mckinsey.com/industries/healthcare-systems-and-services/our-insights/finding-the-future-of-care-provision-the-role-of-smart-hospitals. Accessed 20/4/2022
11. Baig, M.M., Gholamhosseini, H. Smart Health Monitoring Systems: An Overview of Design and Modeling. J Med Syst 37, 9898, 2013. doi:https://doi.org/10.1007/s10916-012-9898-z

Chapter 2
Introduction to Internet of Medical Things (IoMT) and Its Application in Smart Healthcare System

2.1 Introduction

So, firstly we need to know what IoT is and where does it have its application in our day-to-day basis, year 1999 is marked as emergence of IoT by Kevin Ashton where he was presenting his topic were used the term "internet of things" in which he describes how with the help IoT as a technology he will managing the supply chain with the help of RFID tags [1], IoT defined as Internet of things, internet which is now present everywhere so using this network connection can be beneficial so IoT what we do is make such changes to devices which make them possible to stay connected to internet means modifying them with help of some attachment to the device, so that it can be handled remotely for e.g.; – imagine a scenario where we are away from our residence for a vacation and forgotten to switch off certain appliances now it's nearly impossible to go and switch off, what if we have remote access to switch operation off the home appliances present we can easily turn them off and we can save sufficient amount energy and reduce the risk of any hazard due to the overheating of the appliances, Another great example can be like it's cold outside and you are leaving from your office after work now as current pandemic situation it is necessarily have a shower after you reach home for an individual's wellness, it will great if smart water heaters installed in his home so he can remote on and set it so that by the time he reaches his destination he will ready with water.

So, we saw that how these smart devices, yes these are termed as smart devices as they are able to perform task based on the information provided, basically how these IoT devices worked is that it have smart sensors attach to it and all the connected through a circuit, so it sense from the environment from the sensors and the that data is sent to cloud that via network so basically we are converting these real virtual object to have their intelligence and smart so it can perform action on their own when they are directed so, as a connection is established with device than we can control the device from any where and direct them to work as we wish, all

S. Gupta et al., *Blockchain for Secure Healthcare Using Internet of Medical Things (IoMT)*, https://doi.org/10.1007/978-3-031-18896-1_2

possible this wide network present, IoT is just making these device connected by this huge network present which make it possible to pass instruction to these device so they can operate. Now these instructions are sent to cloud where we can connect through are controlling device like smart phones which make them operable.

As in this new era of Advance technology integrating our day-to-day life with these virtual devices will not be shocking fact in next 10–15 years of span time [2, 3] nearly all devices present will be IoT based as if see the growth in employment it is also increasing which make more individuals busy with there task so it make a tedious work to such small task like switch off light, setting up reminders, scheduling meeting, arranging a cab, etc. so IoT devices will form as saviour which can these sort of task just on one simple click, that's why the concept of smart houses are increasing slowly these days. So IoT is next step of evolution for us.

2.2 IoT Related Sub-components

2.2.1 Embedded Programming

IoT gadgets are inserted gadgets, and might be prototyped utilizing commoditized miniature regulator stages, like Arduino, with exceptionally printed circuit sheets (PCBs) created at a later stage. Prototyping with these stages requires circuit plan abilities, miniature regulator programming, and a profound comprehension of equipment correspondence conventions like sequential, I2C, or SPI used to build up correspondence between the miniature regulator and the associated sensors and actuators. The implanted projects are regularly evolved utilizing C++ or C, but Python and JavaScript are turning out to be more well known for prototyping IoT gadgets [4].

2.2.2 Hardware Device

This form the basic unit which are connected with sensors and actuators and are controlling the physical aspects, as we are adding some additional feature of connectivity, we need to add some processing and storing capabilities, which can be done with the help of various microcontroller or integrated circuit.

2.2.3 Security

Security form a major concern whichever sector it comes in IT, as every day we are adding a new device to this large network so we should have a monitor that none of device form a potential attack point, so the need of proper security skills is required so it can ensure that security [5].

2.2.4 Networking and Cloud Integration

This are two most important part of IoT as the number of connected devises and a type of network working. As connection forms the path for communication with other devices and various other application and also utilize the service which are being provided by the cloud. The two important things for proper functionality of IoT are real time data streaming and cloud integration.as the cloud form the base for all basic operation which will be running.

2.2.5 Data Analytics and Prediction

It's becoming important for data to be filtered data and discard irrelevant data, as the number of IoT devises are increasing day-by-day and we need to process these vast queries of data which are being received from these devices.

2.2.6 Machine Learning and AI

It becomes very important to have AI/ML associated with IoT devices as we will receiving a vast amount of data, so it becomes important for developers to have a good knowledge of ML as according to which the model will be trained, irrespective of this technique, technique like data mining, statistics are used to produce predictive analysis and also if required take own decision of data being received [6].

2.3 Architecture of IoT

Basically, we have four stages involved with the architecture of an IoT system, first discuss about Network related things, second deals with sensor data aggregations and digital data conversions, third stage belongs to data processing before delivering it to main cloud storage, fourth and final stage belongs data analysis and stored in form of block of main data (Fig. 2.1).

2.3.1 Sensors and Actuators

First and form the most important stage as it collects data from the environment with the help of sensors, mainly these deals with the physical and digital entities or data like hours of uses, location, etc. e.g.: Sensor to Actuator Flow.

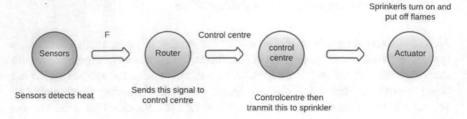

Fig. 2.1 Architecture of internet of things

2.3.2   Internet Gateway

It can be physical device or a software program which work as in transit between cloud and controller. Data aggregation is the process in which data is collected and expressed in such a form so that statistical analysis can be done on that data and all these gathered data are transferred through internet gateway.

2.3.3   Edge Computing IT System

It is more focused on the devices that are being attached to various IoT devices, providing various feature like real-time monitoring analysis and asset utilization and the process data is now comes under more crucial analysis [7], it is also necessary to swap some resources which are not in use as they consume a large bandwidth and it causes an issue with other data processing so proper understanding and dumping is needed (Fig. 2.2).

2.3.4   Data Centre and Cloud

Final layer of IoT architecture which form a facilitator which centralizes the IT operation and equipment, Data managing and analysis is done the most important task associated with this layer is delivering the application required services as requested by the user, and then fed to the servers and this it forms an optimal and secure to store data (Fig. 2.3).

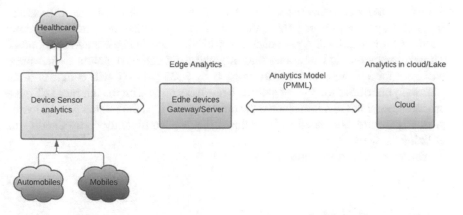

Fig. 2.2 Edge computing system

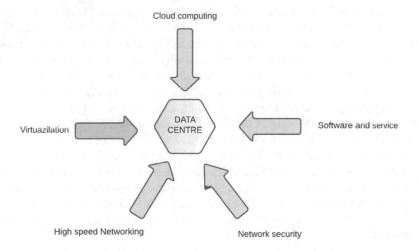

Fig. 2.3 Data center and cloud

2.3.5   *Application of IoT*

IoT is converting this world into a total new dimension with the help various automated functionalities that are being provided by these smart devices our life, if we
look current Greatly hit sector is the healthcare as various feature like remote consultation, reduces the patient to come less in contact and also patient can be handle
with automated devices so which run on the instruction they are instructed and
many more, so these smart devices are the future. As indicated by a study of ABI
Research (statistical surveying and market knowledge firm situated in New York),
there will be in excess of 40 billion gadgets that are associated with the Internet of

things by 2020. According to a new review and study were finished by Pew Research Internet Project, a greater part of the innovation specialists and drew in Internet clients who reacted – 83% – concurred with the idea that the Internet/Cloud of Things, implanted and wearable figuring (and the relating dynamic frameworks) will have far and wide and gainful impacts by 2025 [8]. IoT will comprise of an extremely enormous number of gadgets being associated with the internet. IoT presents some applications that change the entire situation of the human way of living, presently we are associated with machines that are intelligently constrained by us utilizing the web.

Various area of Application of IoT are:

2.3.6   Smart Homes

The fundamental forthcoming of IoT in Home Automation is to construct a smart home gadget that can be constrained by the web. IoT gadgets can be utilized to control and screen different electrical, mechanical frameworks utilized in structures and homes. These frameworks give exceptionally simple working and command over the gadgets. We can handle our home apparatuses (AC, Lamps, entryways, Machines, etc.) [9] by utilizing the web or any product on our Android or some other gadget, regardless of whether we are outside of our home or inside we can look after these webs of things. One of the fundamental advantages of IoT in home robotization is Security; there are a few gadgets which are work for the security of home, similar to Smart Doors, AI Cameras, and the concept of Smart home is turning out to be rocket booming idea and it is estimated that Smart homes will become as normal as cell phones. Which every person wants to have and also this concept will come in vision of various developing countries and government will try to Implement so as meet the competition of various other developing countries among themselves.

2.3.7   Smart Agriculture

With the increment in populace, the interest for crude food is additionally quickly expanding. Accuracy horticulture and brilliant cultivating is new and one of the most amazing use of IoT in the field of agribusiness. The public authority urges ranchers to utilize the new and brilliant procedures of cultivating. The reception of admittance to high velocity web, cell phones, and dependable, minimal expense satellites (for symbolism and situating) by the maker are a couple of key advancements describing the accuracy horticulture pattern. The dirt dampness test innovation gives total in-season neighborhood agronomy backing, and proposals to enhance water use proficiency. There are a few other smart strategies or application gave by IoT to a superior cultivating and horticulture experience like Smart

Greenhouse, Agriculture Drone, Livestock Monitoring, and so on, and these methods assist a great deal with expanding the food creation to lessen the lack of crude food across around the world.

2.3.8 Energy Management

Effective power balance due to the installation of various IoT devices added to the machinery as in near future the rapid increase in population and the rate of finish of minerals like coal, a good control over energy consumption. And it will be like a network of trillions of sensors and devices associated to each other which will together helping in energy management. And setup is done such that all the IoT devices in all machinery are integrated and energy consuming machinery. Smart grid concept is also popular among Energy management with IoT idea behind Smart Grid is that keeping the measure and analyzing the consumer behavior and also consumption of the energy, which will help in both improvement in both economic and efficiency of resources. Smart Grids can likewise recognize wellsprings of blackouts all the more rapidly and at individual family levels like close by solar powered chargers, making conceivable disseminated energy frameworks. These frameworks or applications are extremely valuable for saving power and energy assets by utilizing the assets know it all with the assistance of IoT.

2.3.9 Industrial Internet

The modern web is another buzz in ventures, it is additionally named as modern web of things. Utilizing enormous information, AI, sensors, and programming It engages our enterprises with brilliant machines. Modern web of things holds extraordinary potential for quality control and maintainability. Applications for following products, ongoing data trade about stock among providers and retailers and computerized conveyance will build the inventory network productivity. There are many fields and uses of IIOT in ventures like Digital Factory Facility Management, Production Flow Monitoring, Inventory Management, Plant wellbeing, And Security, Quality Control, Packaging Optimization, Logistic and store network the executives. This application changes the entire situation of the business. With the assistance of IIOT Industries become Smart Industries with better efficiency, quality, approach, and security [10].

2.4 IoT in Healthcare

Amidst this pandemic time remote access of patient and remote treatment of patient helped a lot to decrease the spread of disease as it help in cutting out spread of disease as if less number people come in contact with each other there will be less number of case registered. IoT is to some degree engaged with the field of medical services. It stays the dormant beast of the Internet of things applications. However, with the time and improvement of advancements IOT engage in medical care. As per some examination, IoT becomes huge in the field of medical services. The fundamental intention of IoT in the field of medical services is to engaging people groups to carry on with a sound life. A Smart gadget is made to screen the day by day everyday practice of the individual to give them a legitimate tip as indicated by their day by day way of life. IoT has different applications in the field of medical services from remote observing to sensors and clinical gadget mix. IoT medical services application makes a solid connection among patient and specialist. With loads of professionals, there are a few corns additionally, it isn't not difficult to keep a lot of gathered information of the patients for the Hospital's IT division, likewise this information is imparted to one more gadget so the security of the information is likewise an issue with medical care applications. In any case, with the time IOT is working on in the medical services area, we will see gigantic outcomes in impending years (Fig. 2.4).

2.4.1   Remote Patient Monitoring

In instances of health related crises, for example, asthma or diabetes assault, extreme heart condition, coincidental wounds, and so forth, distant patient checking can be a rescuer. IoT application arrangement empowers interfacing the patient's cell phone application with a brilliant clinical gadget through which the patient can be checked progressively. The associated gadgets can furnish the doctor with a crisis condition related information to the specialist who can then make a move appropriately. Regardless of whether the patient face any basic critical condition, the information gathered through the associated clinical gadget can be utilized to concentrate on the patient's body conduct and indications by the specialist. This information can

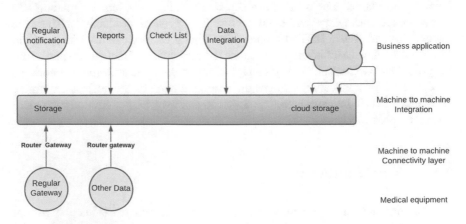

Fig. 2.4 IoT in healthcare

incorporate the patient's circulatory strain, pulse, sugar levels, weight and so forth which is moved and put away on the cloud which can be gotten to by a legitimate individual (specialist or attendant for this situation) and can be examined by them from any distant area as well. This diminishes the opportunities to late deal with of patients just as their readmission rate as issues can be tended to progressively.

2.4.2   Real Time Data Tracking

IoT gadgets play smart role by watching out for the patient's essential details. If there should be an occurrence of a crisis, the gadgets utilize this information following to illuminate the specialists as soon as conceivable with the assistance of cautions and signals. The specialists can make quick moves like sending a rescue vehicle to the patient with the assistance of such cautions like diseases like Heart attack or stroke which show some symptoms so one can help such individual if any signal or indication is there. Patients can likewise help their reports through associated cell phones. IoT helps continuously cautioning and checking along these lines, permitting active medicines with better precision and able intercession of the specialists when required subsequently, guaranteeing total patient consideration.

2.4.3   Connected Wearables

The universe of IoT appears to be inadequate without interface wearables. Associated wearable gadgets not just assistance the clinics and specialists to get data about individuals however they are valuable for people straightforwardly too in light of the fact that they permit individuals to follow their essential body details, for example, pulse, step count, internal heat level and so on Besides, associated wearables can assist specialists with breaking down the patient's information continually in any event, when they are released from the medical clinic office. This is especially useful in instances of patient subsequent visits when they report specific issues in the wake of being released from the medical clinic office. Wearable gadgets are additionally exceptionally supportive for the older as they can send alarms to the specialist if there should be an occurrence of perception of any anomaly in the state of the patient independent of the area. Specialists can make quick moves for the patients with such ongoing alarms, such wearables help in tracking of severe diseases were if patient is not in case to do any body movement the smart wearables can call out nearest hospital and patient can be help out immediately. These are some of the areas were IoT can be used in HealthCare, and there are more too as IoT is a field of growth and every new technology is always welcomed.

2.5   Internet of Medical Things (IoMT or IoMedT)

The sensor-based gadgets that are consolidated with IoT consider reconciliation with portable innovations that are being alluded to as the IoMT (Internet of Medical Things). At the point when the information gathered with these gadgets are joined with electronic wellbeing record (EHR) [11] frameworks, another aspect is opened and numerous conceivable outcomes and utilizations are brought into the world wherein this innovation can assume a urgent part in changing current medical care frameworks, making them more proficient and powerful. In present day clinical arrangements, the IoMT innovation for the most part falls into the accompanying three classifications. Assortment and coordination of clinical information incorporate numerous advances. The IoMT is making this interaction more smoothed out and successful. The information produced from clinical perceptions can be gathered and conveyed as at no other time, saving time and assets by empowering guarantees for what's to come. The use of IoT in medical services is accepting new aspects as IoT answers for medical care rise up out of medical care programming improvement. The utilization of wearable gadgets modified with such programming is becoming standard step by step, as versatile applications and medical care arrangements are becoming open to normal purchasers. To get where the utilizations of IoT in the medical services industry stands, how about we dig into the principle parts of this promising innovation that is bringing a plenty of uses for public medical care.

There genuine worries about understanding security (this escape clause is bounced to be resolve with the blockchain innovation sooner rather than later). Security breaks might bring about genuine information debasement or control, such a hack into medical care investigation might be appalling (blockchain innovation likewise vows to defeat this obstacle). The board of IoT gadgets that comprises of Electronic Medical Records (EMR) framework is a test for current clinical foundations. Action observing turns out to be extremely challenging. Consistence with normalization associations, for example, HL7 and the set up guidelines like HIPAA, FHIR and can turn out to be in fact drawn-out. Norms based interoperable applications stage for electronic wellbeing records like SMART on FHIR might present troublesome specialized difficulties in areas of clinical web improvement. Execution of the HAPI (HL7 API) project and its port execution that is nHAPI can turn into one more snag requiring more detail than medical services area information. The IoT has an exceptionally critical commitment to the Healthcare innovation industry. There have been a few tasks that specialists are dealing with, a handful of them is referenced underneath. Buyer Home Monitoring: Pioneered by a start-up project by a gathering of organizations, the undertaking incorporates observing frameworks like "Qardio" and "AlivCor," permitting purchasers to do their ECG (Electrocardiogram) testing from the solace of their homes without visiting the cardiologist. Wellness Wearables: One of the significant areas of IoT medical services is the wellness business that has created wearables or shrewd clothes like Lumo and OMsignal. There are incredible possibilities that the medical services gadgets in light of IoT will infiltrate a lot further in our lives and the eventual fate of these innovations appears to be extremely brilliant and energizing. IoT in medical services industry can further develop parts, like clinical devices or administrations. It can likewise improve medical services applications, for example, telemedicine, patient checking, medicine the executives, imaging, and by and large work processes in emergency clinics. It can likewise make better approaches for treating various illnesses. The Internet of Things for medical services won't just be utilized by clinics or offices, yet additionally by careful focuses, research associations, and surprisingly administrative establishments.

IoT in medical services industry doesn't remain solitary. All IoT gadgets and their organizations should be joined with different advances to assist medical care offices with changing in a significant manner. As referenced previously, IoT will upset the medical care industry however it likewise needs information, high velocity correspondence, and appropriate security and consistence. 5G will give the super low idleness velocities and portability that the IoT in the medical care industry needs. Thusly, AI-driven arrangements will sort out the information lakes accumulated from an assortment of gadgets. Large Data procedures will utilize such AI calculations to investigate information progressively and settle on basic wellbeing choices. Virtualization will assist with diminishing or dispose of old framework in clinics. IoT is as of now utilizing a large portion of these advances to assist medical care with developing, and this development will just proceed. Sooner than later, medical services and Internet of Things will become indistinguishable, totally changing how we approach our medical care.

- Detecting and transferring modern patient data to the cloud in crisis circumstances, from the emergency vehicle or even from home.
- Clinical gadgets fit for performing self-upkeep. IoT medical care gadgets will detect their own parts, distinguish low limits, and speak with clinical staff and makers.
- IoT and wearables can assist with homing patients and older discuss straightforwardly with a medical care office.
- Telemedicine can be viewed as a "crude" type of an Internet of Things in medical care model. With IoT, a patient can be noticed and now and again treated somewhat through camcorders and other electronic actuators.

This large number of gadgets can speak with one another and at times make significant moves that would give opportune assistance or even save a daily existence. For instance, an IoT medical care gadget can settle on clever choices like calling the medical services office assuming an old individual has tumbled down. In the wake of gathering latent information, an IoT medical services gadget would send this basic data to the cloud so that specialists can follow up on it - view the overall patient status, check whether calling an emergency vehicle is fundamental, what kind of help is required, etc. Accordingly, Internet of Things Healthcare can enormously work on not just a patient's wellbeing and help in basic circumstances, yet in addition the usefulness of wellbeing representatives and clinic work processes.

2.6   Challenges for IoMT

Despite the fact that IoT in medical services gives numerous extraordinary advantages, there are likewise a few provokes that should be tackled. The Internet of Things Healthcare arrangements can't be considered for execution without recognizing these difficulties.

Monstrous contributions of produced information. Having great many gadgets in a solitary medical services office and 1000 seriously sending data from far off areas – all progressively – will produce gigantic measures of information. The information produced from IoT in medical services will probably cause stockpiling prerequisites to develop a lot higher, from Terabytes to Petabytes. Whenever utilized appropriately, AI-driven calculations and cloud can assist with sorting out and coordinate this information, however this approach needs an ideal opportunity to develop. Along these lines, making a huge scope IoT medical services arrangement will take a ton of time and exertion.

2.7   Conclusion

IoT gadgets will build the assault surface. IoT medical services carry various advantages to the business, however they likewise make various weak security spots. Programmers could sign into clinical gadgets associated with the Internet and take the data - or even alter it. They can likewise make a stride further and hack a whole medical clinic organization, tainting the IoT gadgets with the notorious Ransomware infection. That implies the programmers will hold patients and their pulse screens, circulatory strain perusers, and mind scanners as prisoners. Existing programming foundation is old. IT foundations in numerous clinics are outdated. They won't take into account legitimate joining of IoT gadgets. Thusly, medical care offices should redo their IT cycles and utilize new, more current programming. They will likewise have to exploit virtualization (advances like SDN and NFV), and super quick remote and portable organizations like Advanced LTE or 5G.

References

1. Krishna, M & Neelima, M & Mane, Harshali & Matcha, Venu. (2018). Image identification using neural networks. 7. 614. https://doi.org/10.14419/ijet.v7i2.7.10892.
2. Huang, G.-B., Zhu, Q.-Y. & Siew, C.-K. Extreme learning machine: Theory and applications. *Neurocomputing* **70**, 489–501 (2006).
3. Nguyen, G. *et al.* ML and DL frameworks and libraries for substantial and ample data mining: A survey. *Artif. Intell. Rev.* **52**, 77–124 (2019).
4. Kshitiz, K., et al. "Detecting hate speech and insults on social commentary using NLP and machine learning." International Journal of Engineering Technology Science and Research 4.12 (2017): 279–285.

5. S. Kumar, S. Dubey and P. Gupta, "Auto-selection and management of dynamic SGA parameters in RDBMS," *2015 2nd International Conference on Computing for Sustainable Global Development (INDIACom)*, 2015, pp. 1763–1768.
6. Jing Tian, Boglarka Varga, Erika Tatrai, Palya Fanni, Gabor Mark Somfai, William E Smiddy, and Delia Cabrera DeBuc. Performance evaluation of automated segmentation software on optical coherence tomography volume data. Journal of biophotonics, 9(5):478–489, 2016.
7. Ronald Klein and Barbara EK Klein. The prevalence of age-related eye diseases and visual impairment in aging: Current estimates. Investigative ophthalmology & visual science, 54(14), 2013.
8. R. Biswas et al. "A Framework for Automated Database Tuning Using Dynamic SGA Parameters and Basic Operating System Utilities", Database Systems Journal vol. III, no. 4/2012.
9. Sharma, Hitesh KUMAR. "E-COCOMO: the extended cost constructive model for cleanroom software engineering." Database Systems Journal 4.4 (2013): 3–11.
10. Sandler, M., Howard, A., Zhu, M., et al. (2018) Mobilenetv2: Inverted Residuals and Linear Bottlenecks. Proceedings of the IEEE Conference on Computer Vision and Pattern Recognition, Salt Lake City, 18-23 June 2018, 4510–4520. https://doi.org/10.1109/CVPR.2018.00474
11. M. A. Abadi, P. Barham, E. Brevdo, Z. Chen, C. Citro, for example, is one of the most well-known companies in the world. Using Tensorflow, we can do large-scale machine learning on heterogeneous distributed systems.. preprint arXiv:160304467 arXiv:160304467 arXiv:160304467 arXiv:1603044 (2016).

Chapter 3
Internet of Medical Things (IoMedT) vs Internet of Things (IoT)

3.1 Introduction

The term IoT was first coined at the turn of the millennium in the year 1999 in MIT Labs [1] though applications using the Internet to communicate from one device to another existed before that as well. The definition of IoT has evolved ever since and continues to keep on evolving as time is progressing and more utilities are being bundled into IoT due to recent enhancements in the development of newer technologies and computing devices. IEEE document of 2015, available at [2] mentions IoT as "A network of items—each embedded with sensors—which are connected to the Internet". This description is an extremely simplistic way to look at the vast domain of IoT. The IEEE Standards Association has more than 900 published standards as per this document, thus making it evident that one definition of IEEE won't be feasible or practical.

The concept and definition of IoT have expanded over a period of time where various applications of IoT have emerged in the areas like Industrial IoT, IoT for Healthcare, and IoT applications for agriculture to name a few. This concept has further expanded to the Internet of Medical Things (IoMedT), where it is understood that medical devices are connected to each other like in any IoT to ensure the well-being of persons who are under medical care. Multiple authors have tried to define IoMedT based on their understandings over a period of time. One such definition based on multiple inputs by [3, 4] is that the IoMedT is the establishment of the interconnection of one-way or two-way communication-enabled medical devices and their integration to WAN serviced health networks in order to manage and administer the patients' health parameters.

The IoMedT aims to combine reliability and safety features of commonly used medical devices and adaptive, all-purpose and scalability capabilities of the Internet of Things (IoT). It is desired that IoMedT or IoMedT has the capability to address the common problems due to aging of patients and chronic diseases by being able

S. Gupta et al., *Blockchain for Secure Healthcare Using Internet of Medical Things (IoMT)*, https://doi.org/10.1007/978-3-031-18896-1_3

to manage the large number of devices deployed for multiple patients. IoMedT is also made generic enough as it has to deal with a large variety of diseases, thereby requiring heterogeneous monitoring and actuation alerts. As compared to telemedicine systems, which are heavily focused on home-care solutions, IoMedT provides a solution to additional challenges arising out of patients' mobility by providing pervasive monitoring of patients when they are on move even and carrying out their day-to-day tasks [5]. The following sections and subsections highlighted the IoT components, IoMedT components, the comparison between IoT & IoMedT, and finally the conclusion of the chapter.

3.2   IoT Components

The ecosystem of IoT is not restricted to a specific field but it has been expended its boundaries to home & business applications, vehicle automation, healthcare informatics, retail automation, medical, sports, agriculture, and many more [17]. To build an IoT system a large number of components may be considered but there are four fundamental components of IoT devices, namely

 (i) Devices/Sensors
 (ii) Connectivity
(iii) Data Processing
(iv) User Interface

Figure 3.1 depicted the basic components used to design an IoT ecosystem. The following subsections discussed these four major components in detail.

3.2.1   Devices/Sensors

The IoT system starts with extracting the data with the help of sensors. The sensors/devices sense (extract) minute-to-minute information from the devices, it is fixed. Normally, the sensors don't affect by any other disturbing parameters such as rain, sun, wind, etc. but it is continuously gathering information from various sources. The gathered information may have different types of complexities depending upon the various parameter e.g., a sensor for a basic temp monitoring system or a full-fledged multifarious video feed.

Normally, an IoT device may contain of different types of sensor(s) that are used for regularly extracting information to work on gathered data. E.g., a smartphone is a device that consists of various sensors like an accelerometer, camera, GPS, etc. so the smartphone doesn't extract the information from a single sensor but it is regularly collecting data from various sensors. The important and crucial thing about sensors, be single sensor or multi-sensors, is that they regularly extract information from the surrounding area. Figure 3.2 shows different types of sensors that exist in the market used in the healthcare domain along with their expected percentage of usage [7].

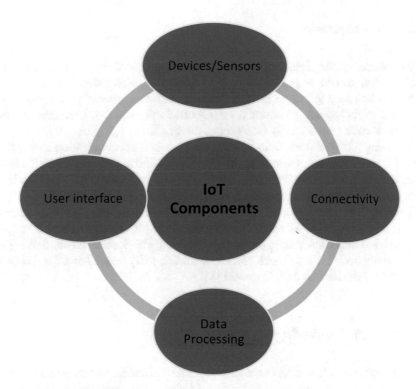

Fig. 3.1 Fundamental components of IoT [6]

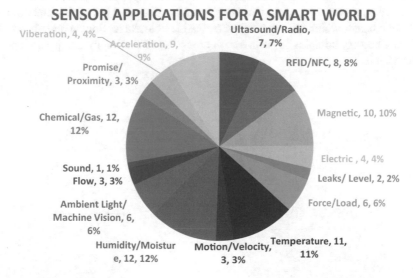

Fig. 3.2 Sensors used in the IoT ecosystem

3.2.2 Connectivity

After collecting a large amount of data from various sources by using multiple sensor, the data should be processed to get significant information from it. So, the extracted data send to various cloud devices for different types of processing and to make this event happen, a medium for transportation is required. This transportation medium is called connectivity (sometimes the Internet).

By using a different medium of transportation and communication as well, the varied-nature sensors can associate with the cloud infrastructure to extract the information from the surrounding area. These types of devices can be Wi-Fi, cellular networks, WAN, satellite networks, low power WAN, Bluetooth, etc.

Different modes of communication exist that have different types of functionalities and specifications. These devices show a trade-off between different parameters such as bandwidth, range, power consumption, etc. So, the selection of a good connectivity option is very much crucial for an IoT ecosystem. Figure 3.3 shows the connectivity devices for an IoT system [8].

3.2.3 Data Processing

The sensors are used to collect the data from its surrounding area and cloud architecture is used to get the extracted data by using various transportation mediums. The gathered data needs to be processed to get significant information from it. To do the same, various software is used to process the extracted data. These devices may work at the primary stage e.g., reading the temperature of a room, AC functioning, and room heater which are working on a considerable range. Somewhere these values may be very complex in nature e.g., object identification by using video/computer vision.

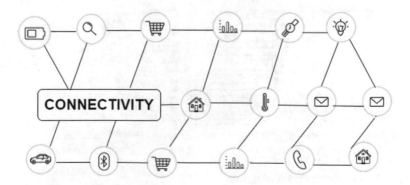

Fig. 3.3 Connectivity in IoT Devices

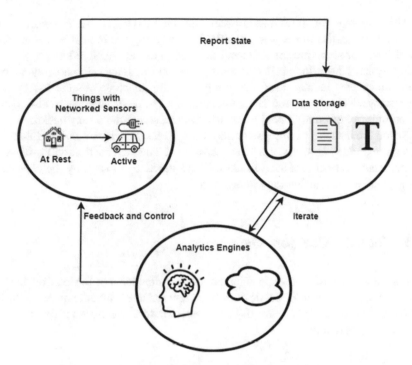

Fig. 3.4 IoT component for data processing [6]

In a few scenarios, user intervention is also necessary to process the acquired data, if the temperature of a room is very much high due to any reason, an intruder in the home but in a hidden area. For such types of scenarios, user intervention is highly needed. Figure 3.4 shows a detailed explanation of the data processing in IoT systems.

3.2.4   User Interface

After taking the data from sensors, the data is transported to the various cloud devices through different-natured connecting media. The extracted data is processed using various software and required hardware. To efficiently process the input data a proper user interface is required to make the available information useful for the end-user. This can happen in several ways such as sending messages/alarms to the user's phone or sometimes by sending emails etc.

In several situations, the software developers design a user interface by which even a naïve user can access, manage, and monitor his own IoT system. There are a lot of real-life examples in our daily life such as a person has installed a camera in his own office or house and by using IoT-based devices he/she can monitor all the events that happened in his office/house through the feed or video recording by a webserver.

The advantages of an IoT-based system are countless e.g., a user can easily detect the defective part(s) in his water purifier by observing the indication on the front panel board or sometimes it will send a message to the registered phone number. Many systems have the ability to perform several actions automatically without (sometimes less) human intervention e.g., washing machine. As the IoT systems have many advantages, at the same time, they have some disadvantages also. Due to the complexity of unawareness of the IoT system, sometime it may backfire.

Several real-world examples of smart ecosystems exist surrounding. IoMedT is also an important example of a smart ecosystem. The next section will discuss the fundamental components used in the IoMedT devices followed by the benefits of integrating of latest technology integration.

3.3   IoMedT Components

This section discusses the various fundamental components of IoMedT devices. As the term defined the IoMedT devices have few common functionalities with IoT devices. Figure 3.5 shows the different collaborators mainly contributing to an IoMedT ecosystem [9].

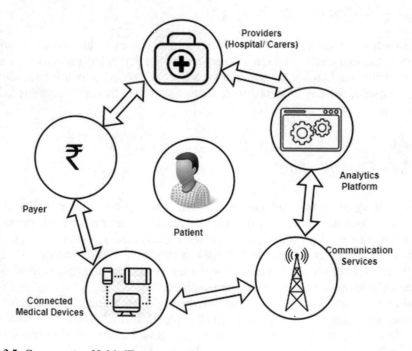

Fig. 3.5 Components of IoMedT ecosystems

  (i) Patient and Payer
 (ii) Connected Medical Devices
(iii) Communication Services (Connectivity)
(iv) Analytics Platform (Data processing)
 (v) Service Providers

3.3.1   Patient and Payer

The main component of an IoMedT system is the patient. The IoMedT ecosystem
starts functioning after getting a person with or without any disease. The input data
is the patient medical history and current medical state of the patient. A payer sometimes called "caregivers" may or may not belong to the patient but is another crucial
part of the IoMedT ecosystem.

3.3.2   Connected Medical Devices

The medical devices are connected through the internet and data sharing can be easily happened in these medical devices. There are many ways to bring connectivity
to these devices. LAN, WAN, and MAN are the fundamental ways to connect the
devices for data sharing.

3.3.3   Communication Services (Connectivity)

Though the healthcare networks are more complex and sensitive when compared
with simple IoT systems. The patient gives also shares their medical information
along with personal data. Sometimes, it will be processed in real time, so the connectivity in medical devices is a major concern. To make it successful IoMedT
needs the best communication services. So the major concern in IoT is communication services which are very similar to the concept of connectivity in IoT.

3.3.4   Analytics Platform (Data Processing)

After getting the input data from a patient, the communication mediums handle the
responsibilities related to communication devices. The data processing units (software) are used to process the gathered information which is similar to the IoT
devices.

3.3.5 Service Providers

The term service providers mainly consist of hospitals, clinics, and carers. Though these service providers don't have direct involvement in smart infrastructure, they provide the basic eminities to the patients where IoT-enabled devices can be installed for further processing.

3.4 Integration of Latest Technology with IoMedT

The functional aspect and components of IOMEDT are depicted in Fig. 3.6. In present times due to the improvements in the area of AI, technology related to sensors, and healthcare informatics, it can be safely said that the IoMedT techniques are the best suitable techniques for taking clinical decisions. In many cases, it has been observed that the decisions taken by doctors, are securely assisted by virtual assistants (VA) and these VAs use AI to specifically learn from patterns and features that lie hidden in the massive pool of healthcare data. This shall be achieved with the help of state-of-the-art algorithms leveraging Deep Learning and especially in the field of radio diagnosis in various hospitals [10, 11]. The abilities of auto-correction can be made available in IoMedT settings which shall be particularly useful to improve decision accuracy based on the feedback loop being fed back into the systems. Text-based mining enabled handheld device-mounted virtual assistants can disseminate the latest and new information from different research databases that include journals and clinical practice reports/case studies for effective patient care [12]. Vitals of Patients can be gauged with help of IoMedT is a continuous activity that can be further used to trigger alerts by tracking events like changing health conditions and patient conditions can be managed as well using the same by taking precautions which are highly essential. Blockchain technology (BT) is another technology for IoMedT which is a sequence of data chunks linked to each on a timeline,

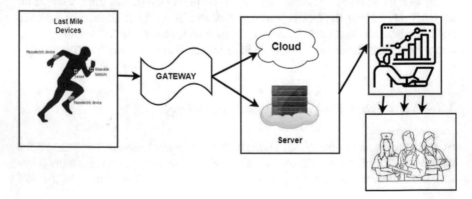

Fig. 3.6 Architecture of IoMedT

vetted by other interested parties in the system. Each newly introduced info-block encapsulates the hash value of the succeeded inf-block and the accompanying data, resulting that making a chain that is progressively prolonged as new info-blocks are inserted at the end of the chain. The data record is effectively monitored by the decentralized compute clusters so that the owners do not belong to a single entity or third party i.e. de-centralized control is the key. BT has positively impacted the financial sector e.g. cryptocurrencies. In the context of IoMedT, BT can be put to use for the integration of three cornerstones of healthcare management i.e. data ownership, integrity, integration, and lastly access control [13, 14]. BT has been showcased that can be possibly used for storing the hash of sensor data to avoid unwarranted alterations and secure the patient's ownership of their data [15]. Blockchain-enabled Supply chains can effectively managed and monitored the drugs and others medical stuffs from the manufacturer to the user by applying edge-enabled IoMedT devices thereby preventing possible mischiefs. Heat control and humidity control mechanisms powered by sensors can be used to manage the physical conditions while supplies are under transportation or inside the storage. Healthcare providers can be provided access to patient records and history on a global ledger thereby benefitting patient management.

On a careful inspection of all the above, one can easily infer that IOMEDT is a special case of IoT where the last mile devices are sensor-enabled smart medical devices, which supply continuous data streams of health-related data. The IoT gateway supplied these streams to appropriate cloud-based infrastructures of computing and storage. The servers act on the data utilizing AI, and DL to create actionable insights, which aid and help the medical staff on the ground. The servers leverage technologies like blockchain while interacting with patient data and creating insights for all parties within a healthcare system.

3.5 Benefits and Challenges of IoMedT

The IoMedT applications can be broadly classified into two categories as mentioned in [12] by the authors. They classify these applications as – Body Centric Applications (BCA) and Object Centric Applications (OCA). BCAs refer interact directly with the human body so that the healthcare devices generate physiological information data to be managed and sent to medical staff for relevant medical analytics. Body non-wearables and wearables of medical nature are famously known cases of BCA. The body wearable devices are the AI-enabled sensing medical equipment, that can be implanted on a human body or be used as an accessory, and another category of smart non-wearables are the sensing devices that are not possible to be worn on the human body. The indoor and outdoor BCAs are two major groups that are segregated based on their environment.

The working behavior of OCAs is not similar to BCAs, the OCAs are indirectly connected to the human body. The OCAs related to the direct solutions of healthcare domains, especially the healthcare services to improve the overall efficiency of the healthcare domain. The hospital management system is an important example of the OCAs. Similar to BCAs, the OCAs are also divided into two groups i.e. indoor and outdoor.

3.5.1 Benefits of IoMedT

The benefits of IoMedT devices are designed devices resulting social life easier, economical healthcare services, improvements in patient outcomes, handling diseases in real-time scenarios, improved social life improvement, better user experiences, improved patient care, an overall reduction in cost, diseases prevention & management, monitoring sensitive health areas such as elder/children, automatic alarm at an initial change in patient health results more lives savvier, on-time medication is on time, affordability, simplicity, patient records management, more energy efficient in terms of time and money, etc. [16].

3.5.2 Challenges in IoMedT

The major challenges in IoMedT devices are a diversity of medical devices, Data privacy, overall performance, data volume, flexibility of medical applications, requirements of medical expertise, CPU efficiency, Memory, network constrained, data sharing, available resources, issues in hardware design and optimization, security, interoperability, and maintaining a relationship between observed measurement and actual diseases, design & implementation of software for medical data analysis, processing of real-time data, predictability, low energy consumption devices, integration, unstructured & diverse data with exponential growth [16].

3.6 Conclusion

The chapter started with the introduction of IoT and IoMedT devices. The fundamental components of the IoT ecosystem discussed, mainly comprises sensors/ devices, connectivity, data processing, and user interface. The details of each component are explained with the help of pictorial representation. Taking into consideration of IoT devices, the components of the IoMedT ecosystem are explained briefly. The major parts of an IoMedT system are patient, payer, connected medical devices, communication services (connectivity), analytics platform (data processing), and service providers. Integration of IoT devices in context with the IoMedT ecosystem was discussed. The chapter ends with the help of explaining the benefits and challenges of IoMedT devices.

References

1. https://www.dataversity.net/brief-history-internet-things/# accessed on 2nd Feb, 2022
2. https://IoT.ieee.org/images/files/pdf/IEEE_IoT_Towards_Definition_Internet_of_Things_Revision1_27MAY15.pdf
3. Mohammad Khalid Imam Rahmani, Mohammed Shuaib, Shadab Alam, Shams Tabrez Siddiqui, Sadaf Ahmad, Surbhi Bhatia, Arwa Mashat, "Blockchain-Based Trust Management Framework for Cloud Computing-Based Internet of Medical Things (IoMedT): A Systematic Review", *Computational Intelligence and Neuroscience*, vol. 2022, https://doi.org/10.1155/2022/9766844
4. S. Goel, S. Gupta, A. Panwar, S. Kumar, M. Verma, S. Bourouis, and Mohammad Aman Ullah. "Deep Learning Approach for Stages of Severity Classification in Diabetic Retinopathy Using Color Fundus Retinal Images." Mathematical Problems in Engineering, 2021.
5. Arthur Gatouillat, Youakim Badr, Bertrand Massot, and Ervin Sejdić, Senior Member, IEEE, Internet of Medical Things: A Review of Recent Contributions Dealing With Cyber-Physical Systems in Medicine
6. https://data-flair.training/blogs/how-iot-works/, accessed on 19th July, 2022.
7. Liu, Xuyang, K. H. Lam, Ke Zhu, Chao Zheng, Xu Li, Yimeng Du, Chunhua Liu, and Philip WT Pong. "Overview of spintronic sensors with internet of things for smart living." IEEE Transactions on Magnetics 55, no. 11 (2019): 1–22.
8. https://www.avsystem.com/blog/iot-connectivity/, accessed on 19th July, 2022.
9. https://www.wowza.com/blog/IoMedT-internet-of-medical-things, accessed on 19th July, 2022.
10. S.E. Dilsizian, E.L. Siegel, Artificial intelligence in medicine and cardiac imaging: harnessing big data and advanced computing to provide personalized medical diagnosis and treatment, Curr. Cardiol. Rep. 16 (2014) 441, https://doi.org/10.1007/s11886-013-0441-8.
11. V.L. Patel, E.H. Shortliffe, M. Stefanelli, P. Szolovits, M.R. Berthold, R. Bellazzi, A. Abu-Hanna, The coming of age of artificial intelligence in medicine, Artif. Intell. Med. 46 (2009) 5–17, https://doi.org/10.1016/j.artmed.2008.07.017.
12. IBM Watson – How to replicate Watson hardware and systems design for your own use in your basement (Inside System Storage), 2015, www.ibm.com/developerworks/community/blogs/insidesystemstorage/entry/ibm_watson_how_to_build_your_own_watson_jr_in_your_basement7 (accessed 7 November 2020).
13. HealthSense: a medical use case of internet of things and blockchain, IEEE Conference Publication, 2019, https://ieeexplore.ieee.org/document/8389459 (accessed 5th August, 2021).
14. J. Brogan, I. Baskaran, N. Ramachandran, Authenticating health activity data using distributed ledger technologies, Comput. Struct. BIoTechnol. J. 16 (2018) 257–266, https://doi.org/10.1016/j.csbj.2018.06.004.
15. X. Liang, J. Zhao, S. Shetty, J. Liu, D. Li, Integrating blockchain for data sharing and collaboration in mobile healthcare applications, in: 2017 IEEE 28th Annu. Int. Symp. Pers. Indoor Mob. Radio Commun. PIMRC, 2017, pp. 1–5, https://doi.org/10.1109/PIMRC.2017.8292361
16. Joyia, Gulraiz J., Rao M. Liaqat, Aftab Farooq, and Saad Rehman. "Internet of medical things (IoMedT): Applications, benefits and future challenges in healthcare domain." J. Commun. 12, no. 4 (2017): 240–247.
17. G. D. Singh, S. Kumar, H. Alshazly, S. A. Idris, M. Verma, and S. M. Mostafa. "A novel routing protocol for realistic traffic network scenarios in VANET." Wireless Communications and Mobile Computing, 2021.

Chapter 4
Application and Challenges of Blockchain in IoMT in Smart Healthcare System

4.1 Introduction to Smart Healthcare and IoMT

The Internet of Things (IoT) refers to an integrated network of physical devices or 'Objects' that use communication to connect knowledge across smart objects [1]. Since Ashton's first reference in 1999, rapid expansion has been observed, resulting in roughly 10 billion linked IoT devices now [2], with a predicted increase to approximately 25 billion by 2025 [3]. Fundamentally, it entails optimizing data transmission and data storage on a cloud security server, from which associated virtual machines form a network to send information and interact across the server [4]. Several advancements have been made on products/devices to make them "smart" using an embedded system that either upgrade existing performance with new capabilities or offers novel activities [5].

Regular inspection of health status in an unusually significant number of patients throughout both pre & post-infection stages is deemed essential during the COVID-19 pandemic [6]. Remote healthcare observation, assessment, and medication via telemedicine offered by IoMT have been widely accepted by caretakers or healthcare practitioners as well as patients. IoMT-based smart gadgets are making a huge effect all over the world [7], especially amid a worldwide epidemic. However, given the great quantity of need, healthcare is expected to be the most difficult sector for IoMT. This organized meta-analysis aims to identify the essential importance of IoMT implementations in developing healthcare systems and analyze the status of data analytics adoption and implementation to demonstrate the effectiveness of IoMT advantages to patients and the healthcare structure [8], as well as to provide a brief overview of the innovations complementing IoMT and the difficulties faced in building smart healthcare [9].

The incorporation and occupancy of the web into the human ecosystem has prepared the way for IoMT services and applications to become a part of the daily routine [10]. The majority of IoMT services operate at the following key levels [11],

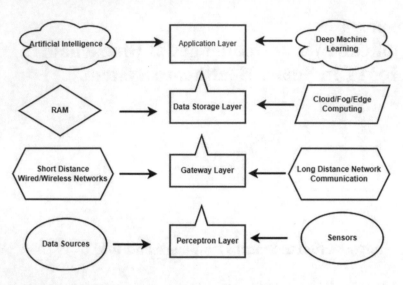

Fig. 4.1 The structure and functionality of IoMT

which combine many innovations, tools, instruments, and platforms that are networked by electronic, hardwired, or wireless communications [12]. Figure 4.1 depicts the structure and functionality of IoMT.

4.2   Perception Layer: Sensor Systems for Data Collection

The perception layer is the smallest unit of IoMT and includes sources of data such as intelligent devices, medical surveillance systems, and smartphone apps that are incorporated with sensing devices such as infrared sensors [13], healthcare sensors, home automation sensors, Radio Frequency Identification (RFID) webcams [14], and Global Positioning System (GPS) [15]. Sensor devices can detect climate changes and distinguish an item's position, characteristics, and magnitude. Further, transform the data into serial communication using a durable, wired, or wireless communication infrastructure that serves as a higher operation channel. These can also memorize and save information for future use [16].

4.2.1   Gateway Layer

As previously stated, devices must be connected to the gateway, which is established through networks that communicate and maintain data either regionally or centrally. Information sharing can occur at various bandwidths and can be either short-range, such as RFID [17], wireless sensor networks (WSNs), Bluetooth,

Zigbee, low-power Wi-Fi, and telecommunications equipment, or long-range, such as cloud technology, cryptocurrency, and so on. Personal Area Network (PAN) connections such as Bluetooth technology, Wi-Fi, and Ultra-Wideband (UWB) or Local Area Network (LAN) connections such as Ethernet and Zigbee are examples of networks [18]. A Wide Area Network (WAN), such as a global system for mobile communication (GSM) that does not have a distributed network but utilizes middleware network services, and WSNs can have sensor nodes, which is useful in some sensors that require limited energy data rate interoperability, can also be used. High-frequency fourth-generation (4G) and advancing fifth-generation (5G) mobile networks are also gaining popularity because they are capable of interacting with a large number of systems at the same time [19]. The enormous information-sharing ability can increase the growth of IoMT applications for healthcare coverage and become its primary driver. The various types of gateways are outlined below.

- **Radio-Frequency Identification (RFID):** This short-range (10 cm–200 m) interaction gateway tag includes a microcontroller and a transceiver capable of detecting a specific sensor in the network, as well as a reader that communicates with the tag via radio frequency to send or receive data as an Electronic Product Code (EPC). RFID does not require an external power source, but it is uncertain and does not function properly with all cellular networks [20].
- **Bluetooth:** Bluetooth is a wireless technology (100 m) that utilizes UHF (ultra-high frequency 2.4 GHz) radio energy to establish a verified, secure, and low-interference interconnection for secure data communication. It is energy-efficient and inexpensive, but even so, it does not serve devices that require long-range information exchange [21].
- **Zigbee:** Zigbee has a mesh network structure, enabling integrated, continuous data transfer between healthcare units. It facilitates data transfer when some of the units are not functioning properly. The bandwidth of Zigbee is similar to that of Bluetooth (2.4 GHz). However, the transmission distance is substantially greater [22]. It is made up of access points, gateways, and a storage facility that allows for data processing and clustering. Zigbee is a low-power wireless technology with a high transmission rate and limited bandwidth [23].
- **Near-Field Communication (NFC):** NFC is a short-range transmission gateway that uses electromagnetic waves among two-loop transmitters that are located close to each other. It functions in two different states based on the use of electromotive force units: passive and active [24]. In the active state, RF is produced, and information is sent without pairing, but in the passive state, RF is produced by only one unit, and the other unit becomes the listener.
- **Wireless Fidelity (Wi-Fi):** Wi-Fi is a wireless local area network (WLAN) with the highest transmission range (within 70 ft). It adheres to the IEEE 802.11 standard and is a popular gateway method used in hospital emergency departments for its quick and effective optimal network capability, increased smartphone compatibility, and provision to enable strict control and security. However, the primary limiting factors are considerably higher power consumption and network unreliability [25].

- **Satellite:** Satellite data transmission is beneficial in rural geographic locations where other ways of communicating are inoperable. The satellite can enhance and send back messages received from the Earth. Approximately 2000 satellites circle the globe, enabling high-speed data transmission and immediate broadband connections. Even though satellite navigation technology is consistent, high-energy consumption is a major bottleneck [26].

4.2.2 Management Service Layer/Application Support Layer-Data Storage

Processing enormous amounts of raw data to retrieve relevant information necessitates the use of tools from the management system or application management overlay that can act immediately using data analysis, control mechanisms, system analysis, and remote access. This managerial layer is responsible for managing users, managing data, and analyzing data. Memory analytics can help to cache massive quantities of data in Random Access Memory (RAM) format to speed up metadata and decision-making. Broadcast data analysis includes real-time or statistical data processing to enable quick decisions [27].

Scalability and flexibility are provided by the application server and its gateways, such as Apache 2 and Flask (Python Web Server Gateway Interface). Database systems such as MongoDB (a NoSQL repository) offer flexibility in terms of the diversity and types of records stored [28]. A Secure Sockets Layer Application Programming Interface (SSL API) is used for strong encryption. Records can be processed directly (fog or edge) or centralized on a remote server. Highly centralized cloud technologies have the potential to be both robust and adaptable. It facilitates the gathering of information such as focused Electronic Medical Records (EMRs) from health apps, IoMT equipment, and smartphone app stores and communicates them to the data center to aid in the therapeutic strategy [29].

However, issues such as excessive information gathering, safety, dependability, visibility, and response time of healthcare information due to the range between sensors and data centers may arise in the future with centralized cloud storage. To address this, a decentralized approach is known as "edge cloud" is being investigated for communication networks and processing. This facilitates data analysis and processing by IoMT sensors and access points (i.e., at the edge). It enhances the throughput of the IoMT machine and diminishes the received data for a centralized location as a result. Another decentralized approach is the "block-chain," which generates independent data sets known as blocks, each with a reliable but particular link. This results in a network governed by patients rather than related parties. The use of the Edge cloud service and blockchain in the healthcare industry is still in its early stages, but it is expected to become an emerging research area in the long term [30].

4.2.3   Application/Service Layer

The application layer's primary jobs are data interpretation and the deployment of application-specific operations. The application layer uses AI and Deep Machine Learning to grasp EMR information and monitor patterns and changes in the gathered information (data conceptual framework) via everyday operational plots to create recommendations regarding diagnosis and/or possible treatments. Aside from computer vision, text categorization, and text analysis, another current state of knowledge includes drug activity design, risk, and genetic mutation interpretation prediction, healthcare outcomes, diabetes, and psychological health management, and estimation of the advancement of heart problems, cardiac arrhythmia, musculoskeletal diseases, neurodegenerative disorders, and malignant and benign tumors [31].

4.3   IoMT: A Boon in Healthcare

The two main drivers driving enormous growth in the manufacturing process and use of medical equipment, especially telehealth surveillance devices [32], are

(a) disorders related unhealthy lifestyles and highly saturated work commitments, and
(b) continued advancements in technology in healthcare tracking devices striving to provide high-quality patient safety at a rapid pace.

Many IoMT innovations, copyrights, and treatment modalities have the potential to enhance health services. The unexpected invasion of COVID-19 has compelled responsible adjustments in the operations, preferences, legal regulations, functioning, and emphasis of nearly all governments worldwide, and has been a catalyst for modernization, advancement, and digitalization, as evidenced by the extensive use of digital media for remote access, telemedicine, and self-health evaluations via wearable technologies [33].

During COVID-19, regulatory agencies such as the American Food & Drug Administration (FDA) granted fast-track clearances and Temporary Use Authority licenses to many COVID-19-related products. For example, Whoop Strap for assessing respiration rate, expendable patches, and diagnostic devices by Philips to identify COVID-19, Scripp's 'DETECT' that can accumulate data from connected wearables, Taiwan's diagnostics and locating design, Eko's electrocardiographic low exhaust valve fraction device for evaluation of vascular difficulties associated with COVID-19, 'Lumify' and other hand-held ultrasound devices alternatives, and AI-CT algorithms for COVID-19 detection [34].

The income from the IoMT industry is expected to be over $66 billion in 2020, representing a 20% rise from 2019 due to the increased implementation of IoMT in the healthcare industry. In the healthcare industry, IoMT has a wide range of applications, the most important of which are remote/self-health monitoring of numerous essential functions such as pulse rate, body temperature, motion monitoring [35], tracking of overall medical problems, nutritional habits, and rehabilitative services of aged people or diseased patients, which leads to an increase in average lifespan and a reduction in mortality rates.

A smart health data system has been created in which various technologies such as MRI and CT may be integrated with laboratory data to enable enhanced diagnosis of medical crises, hence assisting medical personnel in monitoring and making appropriate treatment decisions [36]. It is worth noting that by making hospitals' equipment "smart," expenses might be lower owing to the early detection of irregularities that could impair the accuracy of particular readings from medical equipment, resulting in greater maintenance fees [37].

The rise of IoMT-based smart technologies has also benefited dentistry. Recent innovations attempt to speed up the dentist's job while still providing the patient with comfort and assurance of the process's dependability [38]. AI algorithms, ML approaches, big data analytics, and cloud services are changing dentistry practice. IoMT in dental care includes various present and prospective uses that may become commonplace shortly [39].

As the need for remote treatment grew throughout the pandemic, tele-dental care advanced to the next level. For example, Mouth Watch's Tele Dent services offer a small tele dental platform that allows users to click photographs and send the critical data to a remotely-based dentist for a real-time assessment. In the realm of oncology, machine learning has been developed to precisely measure inflammatory responses in the proximity of oral cancerous cells to give better information on spread and resilience, thus aiding prognostic prediction. Figure 4.2 depicts the various functionalities and components of IoMT.

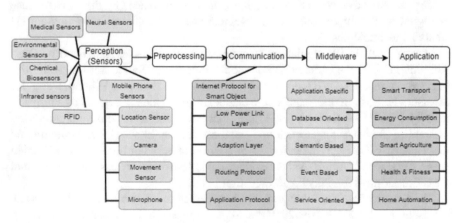

Fig. 4.2 Taxonomy of various functionalities and components of IoMT

4.4 Challenges of IoMT

Several challenges and consequences exist today that must be solved before the widespread use of IOMT, such as security and privacy, information management, scalability and upgradeability, legislation, connectivity, and cost-effectiveness.

- **Privacy and security of data:** Ensuring sufficient cyberspace safety inside healthcare surveillance systems is one of the primary difficulties and challenges in IoMT implementation. The privacy of the massive volume of confidential health information exchanged between devices remains an issue. The safety of healthcare and related data in a cloud-based IoMT ecosystem is provided via a block cipher encryption approach for remote patient monitoring. A SmartCard-based User-Controlled Single Sign-On (SC-UCSSO) healthcare system that protects anonymity while improving performance and security. "CoviChain" employs blockchain technology to solve security and privacy challenges, as well as to prevent exposing individuals' information while attaining more storage capacity [40, 41].
- **Data management:** The capacity to monitor, connect, regulate, and govern knowledge transfer is referred to as information management. Data filtering techniques such as data anonymization and privacy, data transformation, and data synchronization are used to offer only valuable information to the application while concealing unnecessary facts.
- **Scalability, upgradation, regulations, and standardization:** Scalability refers to a medical device's capacity to respond to changes in the external environment. As a result, a massively scalable model ensures consistency among connected things and can perform effectively and seamlessly with the resources available. A highly scalable system is more useful in both the present and the future. Advancements and breakthroughs in IoMT technology have increased the necessity for periodic device updates. This is still a struggle in today's fast-paced environment. The verification of the diverse range of IoMT-based equipment depends on the communication policies and procedures, data integration, and access interfaces, manufactured on a large scale by different manufacturers or distributors, asserting to have followed conventional rules and guidelines during the design phase, has become critical in the healthcare sector.
- Competent authorities or organizations such as the Information Technology and Innovation Foundation (IETF), the European Telecommunications Standards Institute (ETSI), and the Internet Protocol for Smart Objects (IPSO) are required for such certification and standardization. Also, EMR monitoring IoMT devices must be verified. This may be accomplished through the collaboration of researchers, organizations, and standardizing agencies. However, legal hurdles such as the Health Information Technology for Economic and Clinical Health Act (HITECH), HIPAA compliance, and general data protection regulation (GDPR) impede the quick and widespread deployment of IoMT machines.
- **Interoperability:** The standards that support applications developed by various sectors differ. Furthermore, the variety of devices and information acquired from

various sources limits the size of utilization, owing mostly to inter-operator variation. Interoperability is an issue since data interchange between different IoMT systems with disparate characteristics becomes difficult. As a result, standards resulting in their creation become critical, particularly in programs that allow inter-organizational cross-systems. In the IoMT world, the interchange of various types of information generates a large volume of data, and the procedures involved in handling the data, as well as managing the interconnected devices in a compatible manner while minimizing energy restrictions, remain a significant issue.

- **Cost efficacy:** In addition, after COVID-19, economic stress has spread to include a huge number of individuals, businesses, and even organizations, impeding mainstream IoMT adoption. As a result, cost-efficacy has become a major problem that must be addressed. The cost of developing, installing, and using the IoMT system must be reasonable. The IoMT-based system connects a huge number of medical devices and sensors. These have substantial maintenance and upgrade costs that affect both manufacturers and end-users. As a result, the incorporation of low-maintenance sensors with cheap initial setup costs will help in the creation of additional IoMT devices and boost their routine adoption.
- **Power consumption:** Another obstacle preventing the widespread deployment of IoMT devices is power consumption. Most IoMT systems are battery-powered, and once a device is attached, it needs either regular battery replacement or the usage of a high-power battery. The present emphasis should be on developing sustainable healthcare equipment that can generate electricity for themselves or integrating the IoMT network with renewable energy sources, which may also help to mitigate the global energy issue.
- **Environmental impact:** As previously stated, IoMT devices include a variety of biological sensors built-in to execute duties. These are manufactured by combining various transistors that include transuranic elements and other harmful substances that may harm the environment. As a result, regulatory authorities oversee and supervise sensor manufacture. More research should be dedicated to creating and producing degradable devices.

4.5   Benefits of IoMT

Healthcare professionals are indeed stretched for resources, and they may be unaware of how much they're required right now. Patients' real-time tracking via linked devices enables medical professionals to respond quickly to medical crises such as asthma symptoms, cardiovascular disease, and severely low blood sugar levels. IoMT devices capture and transmit crucial health information such as temperature, pulse rate, oxygen levels, body weight, and ECGs to healthcare systems through smartphone applications.

For example, Roche's Eversensing CGM machine is a diabetes surveillance system that may be inserted beneath the patient's skin and enables continual, automated monitoring of diabetes levels in patients, with blood sugar values being reported immediately to the appropriate authorities. Similarly, IoMT-connected inhalers track the frequency of asthma attacks and evaluate the surroundings in real-time to help detect triggers. Real-time tracking is also the cornerstone of telemedicine, which allows specialists to provide precise suggestions to patients without having to examine them in person. Healthcare app development services guarantee the creation of integrated apps that work in tandem with IoMT systems.

Previously, a doctor had to rely on a patient's assessment of how they experienced, but linked medical equipment gives an accurate depiction of a patient's health, allowing for improved condition and treatment. IoMT devices are also being used to monitor patient activities from outside the doctor's office to evaluate a patient's compliance with the doctor's instructions and therapeutic suggestions. IoMT devices assist health professionals in monitoring what occurs after a patient leaves the hospital. Medical equipment such as pacemakers and ingestible tablets provide interval monitoring, which allows healthcare personnel to monitor illness development and define future treatment characteristics depending on a patient's unique living organisms. These gadgets also enable continual monitoring of released patients to expedite recovery and reduce re-admission.

Physicians can now check prescription compliance owing to an ingestible pill packed with sensors that can monitor and alert doctors about how frequently patients take their drugs. The drugs the patient is taking, the precise moment the medicine was ingested, the amount and efficacy of the drug ingested, and the chemical and physical responses to it are all relayed to mobile applications. It assists in determining if the patient is taking the correct dosage of the correct drug at the correct time, as recommended, or if the therapy is successful.

Healthcare solutions give medical practitioners access to real-time information, allowing them to make more intelligent choices and hence offer better clinical outcomes. Scientific proof assessment removes the possibility of mistakes and allows healthcare practitioners to tailor conventional treatments to the needs of the moment. Dedicated processes, more accurate diagnosis, and individualized treatment choices increase the patient's overall experience with the treatment plan.

Patients are now becoming increasingly active in their health coverage as the emphasis shifts to patient-centered care. Fitness enthusiasts are taking control of their health thanks to the rise of healthcare applications that integrate with wearable gadgets. Patients who are well-informed not only strive for optimal health but are also significantly more involved in their care management program and actively participate in healthy choices. Chronic care management is all about driving data from the patient's frequent health check-ups and health evaluations. The Internet of Things has opened up new possibilities for remote patient monitoring. This has the potential to dramatically minimize in-person visits while also allowing clinicians to more properly monitor health markers from a remote location. Data-driven insights and graphs enable healthcare personnel to assess healthcare patterns and determine red flags.

IoMT assists healthcare facilities with improved asset management. Healthcare workers are continuously on the hunt for medical equipment, drugs, and gadgets, and quick availability of resources is frequently vital. Position tracking and indoor geolocation data can assist healthcare personnel in tracking and locating devices within the healthcare facility. Furthermore, IoT devices may monitor the performance of medical equipment and generate notifications if a medical gadget is malfunctioning or requires repair. Folio3 Medical App Development Company assists hospitals in developing outstanding applications that improve investment management.

IoMT devices provide patient monitoring in real-time. Because of reliable information gathering and prompt action by physicians, this minimizes in-person visits as well as hospitalization and readmission rates. When information is recorded and delivered via process automation, human mistakes are eliminated, saving healthcare organizations millions of dollars each year. Some IoMT devices can monitor patients' activities and reactions to medicine, enabling physicians to create individualized treatment regimens rather than spending time and resources on traditional therapies that the individual is not adhering to.

The introduction of IoMT devices has reshaped healthcare. In emergencies, individuals might require medical help from specialists who live a long-distance away. Online consultation with doctors and symptom assessment using video observation, IoMT information, and smart testing are examples of sensor mobility solutions.

The massive volume of data collected by IoMT devices may be used to fuel disease control research. Folio3 EHR/EMR connection ensures that all of this information is saved in a patient's health information. This data, which would have taken years to acquire manually, can assist researchers in understanding illness development and supporting medical research. In certain ways, IoMT devices not only improve the quality of medical services but also pave the way for larger and better therapies.

4.6   Structural Components of IoMT

While IoMT is useful in many ways, there are several connectivity schemes to be aware of. The following are the main considerations if you are on your way to bringing the IoMT platform to reality [42].

- **Ensure security of sensitive medical data**

- Security breaches are the most serious threat to patients, physicians, and device makers. While connectivity in hospitals is advantageous in many ways, it introduces security concerns. Healthcare hacks will have doubled by 2020, costing the sector millions of dollars. Solutions to the problem include: Although medical businesses cannot eliminate cyber risks, they may reduce the risks by implementing real-time data surveillance, undertaking cyber-threat design and simulation, and collaborating with highly secured networking solutions. AI and machine learning are also wise investments for those who wish to anticipate upcoming cyber-attacks and take preventative measures.

- **Take care of regulatory compliance**
- Those participating in healthcare technology innovation must comply with HIPAA, FDA, and other safety regulations. While this is a good thing in terms of security, the regulatory landscape isn't consistent, which might be a barrier in terms of creating or upgrading healthcare equipment and applications.
- Solutions to the problem include: Being proactive is the way to go. Any compliance requirements test on the technological stack should be performed at the planning stage. This can save a lot of time and hassles throughout the installation process. If you choose an IoT platform to connect to, be sure it provides solutions to meet present safety requirements.
- **Enable interoperability**
- Compatibility defines the extent to which devices and systems can exchange and analyze data. Patients and clinicians use various medical equipment to capture various types of medical data, leading to data silos. The lack of interoperability across separate systems is still a problem that must be addressed to fully realize the promise of patient data. Solutions to the problem include: Interoperability between linked medical equipment and technology platforms may be achieved by implementing universal communication protocols for health records, such as FHIR, and integrating open APIs for information sharing.
- **Consider high implementation costs**

- In general, IoMT aims to reduce healthcare expenses, although the installation of such systems is highly costly. Infrastructure purchases, application development, security, and administration all require a significant initial cost, which may impede or postpone IoMT implementation. Solutions to the problem include: They believe that you should only bite off as much as you can chew and swallow. It's sound advice for folks just getting started with IoMT projects. Before the implementation, it is prudent to conduct research, compare pricing for required equipment and technology, and draw up an attainable plan.

4.7   Functional Components of IoMT

Point-of-care testing methods are a diverse range of diagnostic equipment designed to produce findings outside of laboratory settings. They are frequently used in physicians' offices and at home to gather and evaluate samples such as plasma, saliva, blood cells, and so on. Smart pills, also known as smart medications, are miniature electronic gadgets that are packaged in medicinal capsules and feature ingestible sensing devices. Such smart tablets might monitor critical well-being indicators (local pH, temperature, blood pressure), distribute medications to a specific location, and use imaging to effectively diagnose gastrointestinal diseases. Personal Emergency Response Systems (PERS), often known as health warning systems, are specific medical gadgets that employ a help button to summon assistance in emergencies. PERSs can be useful for people who are unable to move and need urgent medical treatment.

Diagnostic and therapeutic wearables are IoT devices and associated systems that have been certified and/or authorized for usage by regulation and health bodies such as the FDA. The gadgets in this category are widely used at home or in hospitals in response to a doctor's recommendation or suggestion. Their primary goal is to improve chronic illnesses and diseases.

Consumer-scale monitors are several types of devices that are used to measure important markers of personal wellbeing or fitness. They have built-in devices that gather and send data whenever a user does physical exercise. Although such devices are sometimes employed for specialized health purposes, the majority of them are not authorized by medical experts. In-hospital equipment and monitors range from massive instruments like MRI or CT machines to smart applications that aid in healthcare monitoring, personnel and supply chain management, and so on.

4.8   Structural and Functional Challenges

The IoMT is a subclass of the IoT, often known as the Healthcare IoT. It is a networked structure made up of medical equipment, software products, medical systems, and services that send actual information via communication networks. A heart monitor that transmits patients' information to the physician's cloud services, where a doctor may evaluate it immediately, is an example of such a "thing" inside the IoMT network.

As per 2018 consulting firm research, the market value of IoMT is expected to reach $158.1 billion by 2022. This is three times what it was in 2017. Almost 60% of worldwide healthcare firms have already incorporated the IoT in some form. There is an increasing need for remote health monitoring. This factor is the result of two developments: an increase in chronic illnesses (especially asthmatic, hypertension, and cancer) and an aging society. According to a USA study, 2.1 billion people on Earth will be old by 2050. Because seniors have greater health difficulties, IoMT devices in conjunction with free software on smartphones can be utilized to assure security and alertness throughout critical occurrences.

Expensive healthcare. Healthcare is getting increasingly expensive, and in some cases, impossible. IoMT technologies have the potential to reduce the cost of industrial services by avoiding major diseases, removing the need for personal check-ups, and offering economical methods of continuous monitoring systems, among other things. According to analysts, the implementation of IoMT can help the US healthcare market save $300 billion in yearly expenditures.

Public health consciousness has grown. With the rise of the COVID-19 epidemic, more individuals have begun to pay closer attention to their health, resulting in an increasing need for effective eHealth techniques and health gadgets to monitor vitals such as temperature, pulse, cholesterol levels, sleeping habits, to mention a few.

In the framework of IoMT, ways to accomplish this such as nanosensors, communication interfaces, and users collaborate to give the greatest health system most effectively and robustly possible. Self-care and early diagnosis are thought to be very important services in enhancing the health care delivery system with the use of IoMT innovations, particularly those that use remote surveillance systems. The collection and analysis of actual information acquired by bio-sensors are critical to a monitoring and control system. Secure procedures and wireless communications are required for data sharing between systems. Security breaches and data breaches are severe issues if these systems are not adequately protected.

4.9 Conclusion

India is a fast-developing nation that lags behind wealthy countries in terms of well-being. To bridge this gap, the medical and healthcare communities are concentrating on the advancement application of emerging technologies. Cloud services, fog and edge computing, AI, wearable technology, big data analytics, and blockchain technologies have facilitated the rapid and safe deployment of IoMT.

The healthcare system has benefited significantly from advancements such as remote monitoring and smart devices, telemedicine/tele-dental platforms, automation, and robotics, which make a significant contribution to preventive medicine by empowering health checks, accurate intervention, strategic planning, and aided living. The ease of use of these patient monitoring gadgets has surpassed the necessity for a medical visit. However, the accompanying issues must be overcome for cost-effective, adaptable, and accurate methods ideal for healthcare demands to gain widespread adoption.

References

1. P. Chithaluru, S. Kumar, A. Singh, A. Benslimane, and S. K. Jangir. "An Energy-Efficient Routing Scheduling Based on Fuzzy Ranking Scheme for Internet of Things." IEEE Internet of Things Journal 9, no. 10, pp. 7251–7260, 2021.
2. Martin JL, Varilly H, Cohn J, Wightwick GR. Preface: technologies for a smarter planet. IBM J Res Dev 2010;54(4):1–2.
3. Gong FF, Sun XZ, Lin J, Gu XD. Primary exploration in the establishment of China's intelligent medical treatment. Mod Hos Manag 2013;11(02):28–9.
4. Pan F. Health care is an area where information technology plays an important role: an interview with Wu He-Quan, a member of the Chinese Academy of Engineering. China Med Herald 2019;16(3):1–3.
5. Farahani B, Firouzi F, Chang V, Badaroglu M, Constant N, Mankodiya K. Towards fog-driven IoT eHealth: promises and challenges of IoT in medicine and healthcare. FuturGener Comput Syst 2018;78(part 2):659–76.

6. S. K. Ramakuri, P. Chithaluru, and S. Kumar. "Eyeblink robot control using brain-computer interface for healthcare applications." International Journal of Mobile Devices, Wearable Technology, and Flexible Electronics (IJMDWTFE) 10, no. 2, 38–50, 2019.
7. Polat K, Gunes S. Principles component analysis, fuzzy weighting pre-processing and artificial immune recognition system based diagnostic system for diagnosis of lung cancer. Expert Syst Appl 2008;34(1):214–21.
8. Esteva A, Kuprel B, Novoa RA, et al. Dermatologist-level classification of skin cancer with deep neural networks. Nature 2017;542(7638):115–8.
9. Wang SJ, Summers RM. Machine learning and radiology. Med Image Anal 2012;16(5): 933–51.
10. High R. The Era of Cognitive Systems: An Inside Look at IBM Watson and How it Works. New York, N.Y.: IBM WATSON. 2012, http://www.redbooks.ibm.com/redpapers/pdfs/redp4955.pdf. Accessed March 20, 2019.
11. Qi RJ, Lyu WT. The role and challenges of artificial intelligence-assisted diagnostic technology in the medical field. Chin Med Device Inf 2018;24(16):27–8.
12. Somashekhar SP, Sepulveda MJ, Puglielli S, et al. Watson for oncology and breast cancer treatment recommendations: agreement with an expert multidisciplinary tumor board. Ann Oncol 2018;29(2):418–23.
13. Wang WD, Lang JY. Reflection and prospect: precise radiation therapy based on bionomics/radionics and artificial intelligence technology. Chin J Clin Oncol 2018;45(12): 604–8.
14. Peters BS, Armijo PR, Krause C, Choudhury SA, Oleynikov D. Review of emerging surgical robotic technology. Surg Endosc 2018;32(4):1636–55.
15. Ye ZW, Wu XH. The latest application progress of mixed reality technology in orthopedics. J Clin Surg 2018;26(1):13–4.
16. Merck SF. Chronic disease and mobile technology: an innovative tool for clinicians. Nurs Forum 2017;52(4):298–305.
17. Willard-Grace R, DeVore D, Chen EH, Hessler D, Bodenheimer T, Thom DH. The effectiveness of medical assistant health coaching for low-income patients with uncontrolled diabetes, hypertension, and hyperlipidemia: protocol for a randomized controlled trial and baseline characteristics of the study population. Bmc Fam Pract 2013;14:27.
18. Andreu-Perez J, Leff DR, Ip HMD, Yang GZ. From wearable sensors to smart implants toward pervasive and personalized healthcare. IEEE Trans Biomed Eng 2015;62(12): 2750–62.
19. Zhang DM, Liu QJ. Biosensors and bioelectronics on smartphones for portable biochemical detection. Biosens Bioelectron 2016;75:273–84.
20. Chan M, Campo E, Esteve D, Fourniols JY. Smart homes – current features and future perspectives. Maturitas 2009;64(2):90–7.
21. Liu L, Stroulia E, Nikolaidis I, Miguel-Cruz A, Rios Rincon A. Smart homes and home health monitoring technologies for older adults: a systematic review. Int J Med Inform 2016;91:44–59.
22. Akmandor AO, Jha NK. Keep the stress away with SoDA: stress detection and alleviation system. IEEE Trans Multi-Scale Comput Syst 2017;3(4):269–82.
23. Yin HX, Jha NK. A health decision support system for disease diagnosis based on wearable medical sensors and machine learning ensembles. IEEE Trans Multi-Scale Comput Syst 2017;3(4):228–41.
24. Estrin D, Sim I. Open mHealth architecture: an engine for health care innovation. Science 2010;330(6005):759–60.
25. F. Pandey, S. Gupta, and S. Kumar. "Information hiding using image steganography – A survey." Journal of Basic and Applied Engineering Research (JBAER) 14, 2014.
26. Redfern J. Smart health and innovation: facilitating health-related behavior change. Proc Nutr Soc 2017;76(3):328–32.
27. Zeevi D, Korem T, Zmora N, et al. Personalized nutrition by prediction of glycemic responses. Cell 2015;163(5):1079–94.
28. White RW. Skill discovery in virtual assistants. Commun ACM 2018;61(11):106–13.
29. Ortiz CL. Holistic conversational assistants. Ai Mag 2018;39(1):88–90.

30. Yang PJ, Fu WT. Mindbot: a social-based medical virtual assistant. 2016 IEEE International Conference on Healthcare Informatics (ICHI). New York, N.Y.: IEEE. 2016, https://www.onacademic.com/detail/journal_1000039757790210_abfe.html. Accessed March 20, 2019.

31. Zhang JZ, Li YK, Cao LY, Zhang Y. Research on the construction of smart hospitals at home and abroad. Chin Hos Manag 2018;38(12):64–6.

32. Li K, Wang J, Li T, Dou FX, He KL. Application of the internet of things in supplies logistics of the intelligent hospital. Chin Med Equipment 2018;15(11):172–6.

33. Álvarez López Y, Franssen J, Álvarez Narciandi G, Pagnozzi J, González-Pinto Arrillagal, Las-Heras Andrés F. RFID technology for management and tracking: e-Health applications. Sensors (Basel) 2018;18(8) pii:E2663.

34. Demirkan H. A smart healthcare systems framework. IT Professional 2013;15(5):38–45.

35. Chen Q, Lu Y. Construction and application effect evaluation of integrated management platform of intelligent hospitals is based on big data analysis. Chin Med Herald 2018;15(35): 161–4, 172.

36. Bakkar N, Kovalik T, Lorenzini I, et al. Artificial intelligence in neurodegenerative disease research: use of IBM Watson to identify additional RNA-binding proteins altered in amyotrophic lateral sclerosis. Acta Neuropathol 2018;135(2):227–47.

37. No authors listed. Oncologists partner with Watson on genomics. Cancer Discov 2015;5 (8):788.

38. Liu JT, Liu YH. Application of computer molecular simulation technology and artificial intelligence in drug development. Technol Innov Appl 2018(2):46–7.

39. Geller NL, Kim DY, Tian X. Smart technology in lung disease clinical trials. Chest 2016;149(1):22–6.

40. Nugent T, Upton D, Cimpoesu M. Improving data transparency in clinical trials using blockchain smart contracts. F1000 Res 2016;5:2541.

41. Kamel Boulos MN, Wilson JT, Clauson KA. Geospatial blockchain: promises, challenges, and scenarios in health and healthcare. Int J Health Geogr 2018;17(1):25.

42. Xiang GY, Zeng Z, Shen YJ. Present situation and development trend of China's intelligent medical construction. Chin Gen Pract 2016;19(24):2998–3000.

Chapter 5
Introduction to Blockchain and Its Application in Smart Healthcare System

5.1 Introduction

Blockchain is created as a chain of blocks wherein each of these blocks has a few virtual facts. Every of the Blockchain blocks has a unique 32-bit complete variety referred to as a nonce that's linked to a 256-bit hash wide variety connected to it [1]. these blocks are connected to each other the use of a sequence of a cryptographic hash feature which links every block to its preceding block. Those three components together ensure protection inside the blockchain.

Blockchain is sent which means that absolutely everyone obtains a duplicate in the case of a public blockchain. So, it's miles very difficult to regulate the information inside the blockchain due to the fact to do so each copy in each area might want to be changed (that's close to not possible) This makes blockchain each dispensed and immutable along with maintaining transparency because the information in the block is not hidden in any way. All of these houses of blockchain make sure the highest stages of security that is why it's so famous in lots of packages that prioritize protection and transparency.

The foundation of digital cryptocurrency is blockchain. The blockchain is a distributed database that contains details of every digital event or transaction that has ever taken place and been shared among participating parties. Each transaction was shown by the majority of system contributors. Each unmarried document from each transaction is included. The blockchain's most well-known cryptocurrency is Bitcoin. When "Satoshi Nakamoto" or an organisation of people with that name published a white paper on "Bitcoin: A peer to see electronic currency device" in 2008, the blockchain generation first came to light. Facts about blockchain technology This makes the transactions in the digital ledger that is distributed throughout the community uncorruptible. Anything of value, such as real estate, vehicles, etc., may be registered.

S. Gupta et al., *Blockchain for Secure Healthcare Using Internet of Medical Things (IoMT)*, https://doi.org/10.1007/978-3-031-18896-1_5

5.2   Working of Blockchain

Bitcoin is one of the well-known applications of Blockchain. A cryptocurrency called bitcoin is used to exchange digital goods online. Instead of using the 1/3-birthday party rule for two events, Bitcoin uses cryptographic evidence to carry out transactions over the internet [2]. Through virtual signatures, every transaction is protected.

5.2.1   Distributed Database

There may not be a necessary Server or other device that stores the blockchain's data. Numerous tens of thousands of computers connected to the Blockchain throughout the world receive the information. The fact that this machine is present on every Node and is publicly verifiable allows for the notarization of information [3] (Fig. 5.1).

5.2.2   A Network of Nodes

A computer connected to the Blockchain network is known as a node. With the help of the buyer, the node is connected to the blockchain. Consumers help with transaction propagation and validation directly to the blockchain. A copy of the Blockchain statistics is downloaded into the system when a computer connects to the Blockchain,

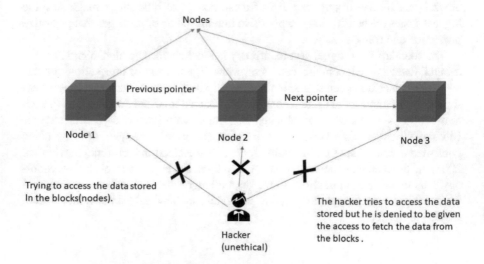

Fig. 5.1 Blockchain basic architecture

bringing the node up to date with the most recent block of information on the Blockchain. The Blockchain node that permits the execution of a transaction in exchange for a reward is known as a miner [4, 5].

5.2.3 Building Trust

Blockchain improves trust across a network of businesses. You don't have to accept people as they are when working on a Blockchain community, not because you can't accept them as people with whom you do business.

Blockchain builds believe through the following five attributes:

- **Distributed:** The majority of the nodes connected to the Blockchain share and update the distributed ledger with each incoming transaction. Since there is no critical server handling the statistics, everything is done in real-time.
- **Secure:** Blockchain is protected from illegal access thanks to permissions and encryption.
- **Transparent:** Since each node or participant in the blockchain has a copy of the Blockchain data, they have access to all transactional information. Without the need for mediators, they may assert their identities on their own.
- **Consensus-based:** All relevant members of the community must concur that a transaction is lawful. Consensus algorithms are employed in the execution of this.
- **Flexible:** The platform can be used to write clever contracts that are entirely reliant on favourable circumstances. Blockchain network can evolve in tempo with business methods.

5.3 Benefits of Blockchain Technology

5.3.1 Time-Saving

No crucial Authority verification wanted for settlements making the process faster and cheaper.

5.3.2 Cost-Saving

A blockchain community cuts costs in a variety of ways. The 0.33-celebration verification is not needed. Direct asset percentages are possible for people [5, 6]. There are fewer intermediaries. Since each player has a copy of the shared ledger, transaction efforts are kept to a minimum.

5.3.3   Tighter Security

No person can mood with Blockchain records as it shared amongst thousands and thousands of players. The device is secure against cybercrimes and Fraud.

5.4   Application of Blockchain

Some applications of Blockchain in the real world are as follows:

- Asset Management
- Cross-Border Payments
- Healthcare
- Cryptocurrency
- Birth and Death Certificates
- Online Identity Verification
- Internet of Things
- Copyright and Royalties

5.4.1   Asset Management

Blockchain performs a big part inside the monetary world and it is no different in asset management. In trendy terms, asset management includes the dealing with and exchange of various assets that a person may additionally own inclusive of fixed earnings, actual property, equity, mutual budget, commodities, and different opportunity investments. Everyday trading tactics in asset control can be very costly, mainly if the buying and selling entails a couple of international locations and pass border bills. In such conditions, Blockchain may be a big assist because it eliminates the needs for any intermediaries including the dealer, custodians, agents, settlement managers, and so forth. Instead, the blockchain ledge presents a simple and obvious system that gets rid of the probabilities of error [7, 8].

5.4.2   Cross-Border Payments

Have you ever tried to make go-border bills in distinctive currencies from one united states of America to any other? this will be a protracted complicated technique and it could take many days for the cash to reach at its vacation spot. Blockchain has helped in simplifying these move border bills via supplying stop-to-end remittance services with none intermediaries. There are numerous remittance groups that provide Blockchain offerings which may be used to make international remittances inside 24 hours.

5.4.3 Healthcare

Blockchain may have a massive effect on healthcare the use of clever contracts. These clever contacts imply that a contract is made between two parties without needing any middleman. All the parties involved in the contract realize the agreement info and the contract is implemented routinely whilst the agreement conditions are met. This will be very beneficial in healthcare carrying private fitness information can be encoded thru Blockchain so they may be simplest handy to number one healthcare vendors with a key. They also assist in upholding the HIPAA privacy Rule which ensures that affected person records is confidential and now not available to anybody [8–10].

5.4.4 Cryptocurrency

Perhaps one of the maximum famous applications of Blockchain is in Cryptocurrency. Who hasn't heard about bitcoin and its insane popularity? one of the many benefits of cryptocurrency the use of blockchain because it has no geographical boundaries. So crypto cash may be used for transactions everywhere in the global. The only critical element to keep in thoughts is alternate quotes and that people may additionally lose some money in this method. But this **selection** is a great deal better than nearby fee apps along with Paytm in India that are only relevant in a selected U.S. or geographical region and can't be used to pay money to human beings in other international locations.

5.4.5 Birth and Death Certificates

There are many human beings inside the global who don't have a valid birth certificate in particular inside the poorer international locations of the world. in keeping with UNICEF, one-0.33 of all the children beneath the age of 5 don't have a birth certificate. And the trouble is just like dying certificates as well. However, Blockchain can assist in solving this problem by using developing a cozy repository of start and dying certificate which might be demonstrated and can handiest be accessed by means of the legal people [10].

5.4.6   Online Identity Verification

It is not viable to complete any financial transactions on line without on-line verification and identification. And that is authentic for all the possible provider carriers any person might have in the economic and banking enterprise. But, blockchain can centralize the web identification verification process in order that customers only want to verify their identification once using blockchain after which they are able to percentage this identity with whichever provider issuer they need. Users additionally have the choice to pick their identification verification techniques along with person authentication, facial popularity, etc.

5.4.7   Internet of Things

Internet of things is a community of interconnected devices that can interact with others and acquire records that may be used for gaining beneficial insights. Any device of "things" will become IoT once its miles linked [11]. The maximum not unusual instance of IoT is perhaps the clever domestic wherein all the house appliances inclusive of lights, thermostat, air conditioner, smoke alarm, etc. may be linked collectively on an unmarried platform. However where does Blockchain come into this? properly, Blockchain is needed for presenting safety for this massively dispensed device. In IoT, the safety of the device is simplest as properly as the least secured device that is the vulnerable hyperlink. Right here Blockchain can make sure that the records acquired by the IoT gadgets are secure and most effective visible to relied on parties.

5.4.8   Copyright and Royalties

Copyright and royalties are a massive issue in innovative sectors like tune, films, and so on. those are inventive mediums and it doesn't sound like they have got any hyperlink with Blockchain. but this technology is pretty crucial in ensuring security and transparency in the creative industries. There are many instances wherein song, films, art, and many others. is plagiarized and due credit score isn't given to the authentic artists. This can be rectified the use of Blockchain which has a detailed ledger of artist rights. Blockchain is also transparent and may provide a relaxed report of artist royalties and deals with massive production corporations. The price of royalties can also be managed using virtual currencies like Bitcoin [12].

5.5   Application of Blockchain in Smart Healthcare

This is one area in which blockchain technology can help the situation. It is capable of a wide range of tasks, including handling epidemics and providing secure patient data encryption. As a pioneer in this field, Estonia began utilising blockchain technology in healthcare in 2012. Currently, blockchain is used to retain 100% of prescription statistics, 95% of fitness records, and 100% of all healthcare billing. DLT can be used in a variety of healthcare settings, however not all healthcare-related interests are transaction-related. Public blockchains cannot, however, be utilised to store personally identifiable information or medical records because the information contained therein is widely accessible. This transparency mandates that companies recollect privacy problems to make sure blanketed health records (PHI) [13, 14]. Second, although it provides built-in protection against some types of threats, blockchain technology is susceptible to a few. The blockchain code makes it vulnerable to social engineering, 0-day attacks, and errors. Because of this, extreme care must be used when using statistics in the healthcare industry. Due to the immutability of its facts, blockchain technology should no longer be applied arbitrarily in the healthcare industry. Large files or those that often interchange can be excluded. Any personal information should be kept off the chain. "With new regulations on the rise", such as the general data protection law (GDPR), in conjunction with policies that have been around for more than a decade, including with HIPAA [11], DLT specialists note that these regulations are particularly important. When processing any form of PHI, patient privacy is now a well-known concern. The benefits of using blockchains over traditional methods of healthcare database management systems include decentralised management, immutable databases, records provenance, traceable information, strong records, availability of facts to any legal person, while also keeping it out of the hands of unauthorised users with the aid of encryption. There are five main areas where blockchains in healthcare could be used:

Coping with digital scientific record (EMR) data

- Safety of healthcare records
- Personal fitness report statistics management
- Point-of-care genomics control
- Electronics health statistics management

Some specific applications include the following.

5.5.1   Research

The automatic updating and sharing of clinical information on a certain patient are currently only possible inside a single employer or group of businesses thanks to digital health statistics. If the data was prepared in such a way that only information that was not PHI or personally identifiable information (PII) was included in the hard and fast of data at the top layer of the blockchain, this might be prolonged [14].

This would make it possible for researchers and other businesses to access this vast array of data, which includes cohorts of countless thousands of patients. Having access to such a wealth of information might significantly advance public health reporting, safety occasion and bad event reporting, and medical research.

5.5.2   Seamless Switching of Patients Between Providers

Through a shareable personal key, the identical data on the blockchain should make it simple for individual patients to unblock and share their fitness records with other businesses or groups. This may facilitate exclusive customers' collaboration and interoperability using fitness records technology (HIT).

5.5.3   Faster, Cheaper, Better Patient Care

Blockchain can create an unmarried machine for saved, continuously updated, heath information for cozy and fast retrieval by using legal customers. Via averting miscommunication among exceptional healthcare experts worried in worrying for the equal affected person, innumerable errors can be averted, quicker analysis and interventions end up viable, and care may be customized to every patient.

5.5.4   Interoperable Electronic Health Records

The blockchain should offer a single transaction layer where businesses may publish and share data through a single secure device by storing a specific set of standardised data on the chain, with private encrypted linkages to one at a time saved data as well as radiography or other images. The adoption of uniform authorisation mechanisms and intelligent contracts can significantly promote seamless communication (Fig. 5.2).

5.5.5   Data Security

Over 176 million data breaches involving healthcare information occurred between 2009 and 2017. Fitness records may be much better protected thanks to the secure features of the blockchain. Each person has a personal key that can only be used as

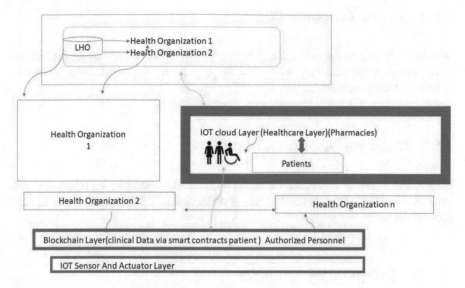

Fig. 5.2 IoT and blockchain in E-healthcare

and for the time necessary, as well as a public identification or key. Additionally, the desire to attack every user in order to obtain personal data may limit hacking. Blockchains can consequently provide a health records audit path that cannot be changed.

5.5.6   Mobile Health Apps and Remote Monitoring

With the advancement of technology, cell health packages are becoming more and more important. In this context, it was found that electronic medical records (EMRs) were stored carelessly in a blockchain network and that the information could be quickly supplied to medical staff in addition to being accessible for self-monitoring and domestic care. This region is particularly vulnerable to malware, but especially root exploits that could give the hacker access to the target's private key.

5.5.7   Tracing and Securing Medical Supplies

Blockchain can put your mind at ease and clearly identify the medicinal component's route. Additionally, it might offer monitoring of the labour costs and carbon emissions incurred during the production of these products.

5.5.8   Health Insurance Claims

Due to its ability to provide scientific events as they occurred without the risk of later changing the statistics for fraudulent objectives, the blockchain is ideally suited to claim processing.

5.5.9   Tracking Diseases and Outbreaks

Blockchain's unique capabilities can aid with real-time disease reporting and the investigation of illness patterns that may reveal a disease's origin and parameters for propagation.

5.5.10   Safeguarding Genomics

Blockchain can help you with this or even offer a virtual market where scientists may buy genomic statistics for their research. This might discourage middlemen who charge high prices and promote secure selling. Healthcare blockchain applications are still in their infancy. Ethereum and Hyperledger fabric are two examples of blockchain generation frameworks that are currently being used on a very limited scale. Blockchain services may be utilised to enhance the management of medical records if they had increased blockchain security and architecture that encouraged synchronised transactions.

5.6   Conclusion

Blockchain is an exceedingly new generation that is nonetheless no longer sizable in all industries however it's miles slowly gaining greater momentum. Once Blockchain turns into bigger, it could end up a powerful tool for the democratization of information as a way to inspire transparency and moral enterprise approaches. And the programs of Blockchain within the international are handiest growing with the result of faster transactions, greater transparency, and protection as well as decreased prices. Who knows, Blockchain may additionally exchange the arena within the destiny!

References

1. Krishna, M & Neelima, M & Mane, Harshali & Matcha, Venu. (2018). Image identification using neural networks. 7. 614. https://doi.org/10.14419/ijet.v7i2.7.10892.
2. Huang, G.-B., Zhu, Q.-Y. & Siew, C.-K. Extreme learning machine: Theory and applications. *Neurocomputing* **70**, 489–501 (2006).
3. Nguyen, G. *et al.* ML and DL frameworks and libraries for substantial and ample data mining: A survey. *Artif. Intell. Rev.* **52**, 77–124 (2019).
4. Kshitiz, K., et al. "Detecting hate speech and insults on social commentary using NLP and machine learning." International Journal of Engineering Technology Science and Research 4.12 (2017): 279–285.
5. S. Kumar, S. Dubey and P. Gupta, "Auto-selection and management of dynamic SGA parameters in RDBMS," 2015 2nd International Conference on Computing for Sustainable Global Development (INDIACom), 2015, pp. 1763–1768.
6. Jing Tian, Boglarka Varga, Erika Tatrai, Palya Fanni, Gabor Mark Somfai, William E Smiddy, and Delia Cabrera DeBuc. Performance evaluation of automated segmentation software on optical coherence tomography volume data. Journal of biophotonics, 9(5):478–489, 2016.
7. Hitesh Kumar Sharma; Anuj Kumar; Sangeeta Pant; Mangey Ram, "Artificial Intelligence, Blockchain and IoT for Smart Healthcare," in *Artificial Intelligence, Blockchain and IoT for Smart Healthcare*, River Publishers, 2022, pp. i–xvi.
8. Hitesh Kumar Sharma; Anuj Kumar; Sangeeta Pant; Mangey Ram, "1 Introduction to Smart Healthcare and Telemedicine Systems," in Artificial Intelligence, Blockchain and IoT for Smart Healthcare, River Publishers, 2022, pp. 1–12.
9. Hitesh Kumar Sharma; Anuj Kumar; Sangeeta Pant; Mangey Ram, "2 Advanced Technologies Involved in Smart Healthcare and Telemedicine Systems," in Artificial Intelligence, Blockchain and IoT for Smart Healthcare, River Publishers, 2022, pp. 13–24.
10. Hitesh Kumar Sharma; Anuj Kumar; Sangeeta Pant; Mangey Ram, "3 Role of Artificial Intelligence, IoT and Blockchain in Smart Healthcare," in Artificial Intelligence, Blockchain and IoT for Smart Healthcare, River Publishers, 2022, pp. 25–36.
11. Ronald Klein and Barbara EK Klein. The prevalence of age-related eye diseases and visual impairment in aging: Current estimates. Investigative ophthalmology & visual science, 54(14), 2013.
12. R. Biswas et al. "A Framework for Automated Database Tuning Using Dynamic SGA Parameters and Basic Operating System Utilities", Database Systems Journal vol. III, no. 4/2012.
13. Sharma, Hitesh KUMAR. "E-COCOMO: the extended cost constructive model for cleanroom software engineering." Database Systems Journal 4.4 (2013): 3–11.
14. M. A. Abadi, P. Barham, E. Brevdo, Z. Chen, C. Citro, for example, is one of the most well-known companies in the world. Using Tensorflow, we can do large-scale machine learning on heterogeneous distributed systems.. preprint arXiv:160304467 arXiv:160304467 arXiv:160304467 arXiv:1603044 (2016).

Chapter 6
Digital Medical Records (DMR) Security and Privacy Challenges in Smart Healthcare System

6.1 Introduction

To fully appreciate the complexity of the expanding electronic health record systems, it helps to be aware of the past, present, and future needs of the health information system. Paper or electronic medical records serve as communication tools for clinical decision-making, service coordination, evaluation of the quality and efficacy of care, research, legal protection, education, accreditation, and regulatory processes. This is a business record for a medical system that was created as part of routine business. The document must be authenticated, and the entry on a handwritten document must be legible. In the past, medical records were merely a paper repository for data that was analyzed or used for administrative, clinical, financial, and research purposes. It could only be accessed by one user at a time and had very strong accessibility restrictions. Manually updating paper-based records caused a delay of more than 1–6 months in finishing the records. As a result of the amount of paper clogging up other areas, the majority of the medical record departments were housed in the building's basement. The doctor oversaw the nursing and documentation process and provided his consent for the sharing of the information. Patients very infrequently review their medical records [1]. Electronic medical records (EHR), according to the Centers for Medicare and Medicaid Services (CMS), are "an electronic representation of a patient's medical history that the provider retains throughout time and uses for all relevant clinical management needs." Data that could be presented include: "demographics, medical records, issues, prescriptions, vital signs, medical history, immunity, test results, and radiation for the individual's care at a certain provider". The next step in the evolution of healthcare is the use of electronic medical records, but before taking this step, it is important to thoroughly comprehend the cybersecurity measures involved [2]. Due to the high level of secrecy of the data stored in EHRs, a few protections are offered under the Health

Insurance Portability and Accountability Act (HIPAA) and the Health Insurance Portability and Accountants (HITECH) Act.

Internet of Things (IoT) constitutes a huge number of sensor nodes, and communication hardware including powerful base stations, servers, or cloud storage which are connected via the internet. Sensor nodes are usually small, have one or more sensors, and a microcontroller, are not so expensive, are low performance, and battery operated wireless computing devices. These nodes collect the data, transmit them over the internet and store it on servers/cloud for processing and analysis. The early use of IoT was in military applications, but nowadays IoT is also being deployed in almost all the industrial and civilian domains such as agriculture, health, retail market, logistics, habitat monitoring, and many other areas. In applications that require the secure transmission of sensitive data to the base station over several hops, it is also seeing extensive use. Because these applications employ space as a communication medium, it is quite simple for an enemy to intercept the information. Hence, they access the information, and new malicious sensor nodes can enter the existing network. They can therefore harm the security of the complete network. Akyildiz et al. [1] introducing security mechanisms is very essential and it normally involves establishing cryptographic methods. These cryptographic methods require comparatively large memory and consume high power while processing and communicating the information. IoT networks become more vulnerable to security threats because of the broadcasting nature of the transmission medium. Shamir et al. [29] say these networks have added vulnerabilities because sensor nodes are frequently installed in harsh or hazardous environments where they are also exposed to physical threats and technical threats.

In the military and other sensitive applications, IoT networks are used to handle crucial information. Due to this, many challenges need to be considered to protect and safeguard the crucial information traveling between these nodes [28]. Further, as the sensor nodes are mainly wireless devices, they have a limited amount of memory and other resources. They also have limited power and computing abilities. So implementing complex security techniques also poses challenges. Some of the major security requirements are now discussed by Ilyas et al. [13].

- Confidentiality: Confidentiality is the assurance that sensitive information is well protected and not disclosed to unapproved parties. This criterion in IoT networks makes sure that no adversary who may eavesdrop on the communication channel learns about the information traveling

- (i) Between the sensor nodes or (ii) between the sensor nodes and the base station.
- Integrity: There are chances that the information gets distorted while traveling over insecure IoT networks. This lack of integrity in the information gives rise to many other challenges as the outcomes of utilizing erroneous information are normally devastating.
- Availability: This requirement ensures that both services, as well as the information, could be accessed at any instant of time and also whenever they are needed. In IoT networks, denial of service attacks results in non-availability of the sys-

tem or network that impacts the operations of many sensitive applications, Hence Yick et al. [36] say it becomes essential to ensure the availability of the IoT network and provide solutions to immediately fill in the gap created by deactivating specific sensor node or base station by assigning its responsibilities to some other similar sensor nodes in the network

- Authentication: Authentication methods are used to confirm the identity of users. These methods distinguish between legitimate users and illegitimate users. In the case of IoT networks, every sensor node and communication hardware such as the base station needs to confirm that the data it has received is in reality sent by a trusted source. An adversary may trick the sensor node or base station into a legitimate source and traps them to accept false data. If false data happens to get into the network, then the network behavior could change and may produce unexpected results [5].

As the IoT networks are quite complex, some additional security requirements must also be kept in mind while designing these networks. These requirements as given by Tan et al. [30] and Batty et al. [3] are now discussed below and are also shown in Fig. 6.1.

- Mutual Authentication: Any two systems belonging to an IoT network must authenticate each other (for instance user and cloud) by giving their identity and verifying each other.
- Reliability and Responsibility: In IoT applications such as smart cities one must ensure the availability of reliable information 24 × 7 and proper access control

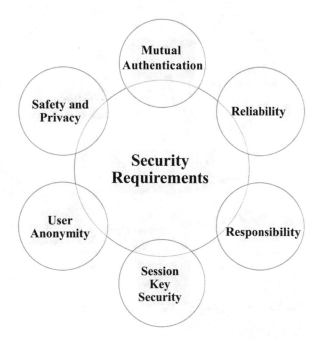

Fig. 6.1 Additional security requirements of IoT networks

mechanisms to provide services to authorized users. It, therefore, becomes the responsibility of IoT networks to ensure this.

- Session Key Security: It is established during the communication between the two entities and it must be ensured that it is secure. While designing IoT networks, it must be ensured that the session key is not compromised.
- User anonymity: The identification of the user must be kept secret and must not leak in case of security threats. The anonymity of the user during the message transmission must be of high priority.

6.2   Possible Security Attacks in DMR Internet of Things Networks

Figure 6.2 depicts the types of attacks possible in IoT networks. These are now explained in the following section.

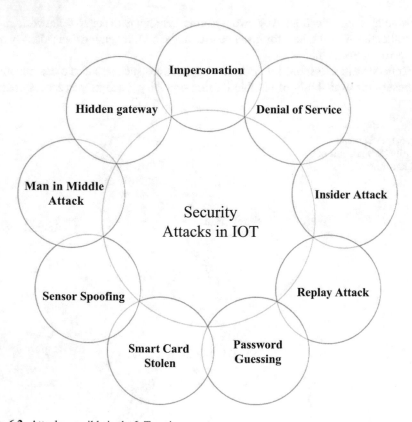

Fig. 6.2 Attacks possible in the IoT environment

- Denial of service attack (DoS): This inactivates the sensor node or base station that provides services to the user in an IoT network [15]. In this attack, an adversary sends several requests to the sensor node or base station to slow down or disable it and thereby slowing down or shutting down the IoT network.
- Insider attack: Here an inside who is a legitimate and authentic user accesses the IoT network in an unauthorized way. He captures the crucial data in the IoT network or present in the server and misuses it [25].
- Replay attack: Here, the adversary either delays or replays the data while the data is traveling in the IoT network [20].
- Password guessing attack: It can be of two types viz. (i) offline attack, in which eavesdropping of the communication channel and capturing of the information during transmission takes place, and (ii) online attack, in which an adversary uses brute force method and tries a large number of user names and password combinations to try logging into the IoT network to capture the information [26].
- Stolen/lost smart card: The adversary performs power analysis to decode the information stored in the smart card [7].
- Man in the middle attack (MIMA): Here, an adversary penetrates the communication path between two parties. He monitors the secret information being transmitted [2].
- Impersonation attack: Mustafa et al. [24] say when two transmitters (one legitimate and the other illegitimate) send the information to the receivers. The illegitimate transmitter tries to spoof the information at the receiver. Thus, the receiver is confused if the sender is a legitimate user or not.
- Hidden gateway attack: Here an adversary login to the application, and remotely change and update the information [7, 8]. To avoid such attacks, an authentication scheme and key exchange method are needed.

6.3 Security Schemes and There Challenges in DMR

Numerous access control strategies are presented in the literature to protect communication over IoT networks made up of sensor nodes, base stations, clouds, and users. Zhou et al. [37] proposed one such method based on Elliptic Curve Cryptography (ECC) that enables new sensor nodes to dynamically join the network [17]. It permits new sensor nodes to establish keys with their neighbors to carry out secure communication and each sensor node is capable of sustaining a time interval (called tolerance time) before it gets compromised [21]. The concept of bootstrap time is also proposed in the authentication mechanism. Using a Novel Access Control Scheme, Huang [11] (NACP). ECC and a hash chain form the basis of NACP. For sensor nodes with limited power and resources, NACP is extremely effective. Because NACP uses a dynamic access control system, no changes are required to the current sensor nodes' broadcasting data when a new sensor node joins the network. Huang's NACP is resistant to forgery and replay attacks. Huang's

NACP strategy decreases both the quantity of I calculations and (ii) communications between two sensor nodes when compared to Zhou et al.'s [37] scheme.

Each sensor node in the H. Hwang and Liu [11] suggested approach completes five one-way hash functions and four bit-wise XOR operations to accomplish mutual authentication. By avoiding steps like modular exponentiation and inverse computing, it uses the shared key establishment technique to lower operational costs. The Enhanced Novel Access Control Scheme (ENACP) developed by Kim and Lee [16] adds a step known as hash chain renewal and facilitates mutual authentication. The authors claim that ENACP is secure against attacks like replay, new node masquerading, and lack of hash chain renewability. Lee and Shin [18] suggested a Practical Access Control Scheme (PACP) for securing IoT networks by discussing the discrepancies in Huang's scheme. According to them, NACP [10] is not dynamic in the real sense. In addition, the authentication mechanism by using a hash chain requires an enormous amount of both communication cost and memory overhead. In contrast to ENACP, Hwaseong's scheme simply uses hash operations instead of a hash chain, which makes their scheme more realistic in terms of communication overhead and computation costs. It may be mentioned here that this scheme does not provide for a permanent network lifetime.

Shen et al. [29] deliberated that ENACP [18] is not completely error-free even though it has significant improvement over NACP. In the authentication phase and also in the key establishment phase, an intruder can intercept a random number that belongs to the base station quite easily. He also gets to know hash operation in the initialization phase. The intruder blocks both the random number and hash operation. He then resubmits after altering the random number and hash function. In this case, the sending node cannot transmit the authentication to the receiving node which then considers the sending node as an illegitimate node. This is because the verification could not take place because of a modified random number that was submitted. In IoT networks, Huang et al.'s New Design of Access Control (NDAC) was introduced in 2011 [12] and inhibits key establishment during the authentication process. Lee and Shin [19] presented PACPs, or Practical Access Control Schemes, in 2012. It has been shown that PACPs are more secure against all threats and have lower communication overhead and computation costs than other approaches [6].

In the literature, many schemes based on a symmetric key [20] or an asymmetric key [26] have been given. Symmetric key public cryptography is used where either multicasting or broadcasting type of communication is prevalent. Most of the time RSA algorithm and ECC [21] are deployed for the sensor nodes of IoT networks. The number of the authentication schemes in this category is given in [12–16].

Some smart card-based user authentication techniques have been proposed. A user authentication method for ad hoc sensor networks, which are often wireless when utilized for IoT, was suggested by Turkanovic et al. in 2014 [31]. The system enables a distant user to generate a key to start a session and carry out authentication. But this system does not allow for user and IoT gateway mutual authentication. Their authentication model that has four steps does not ensure anonymity and privacy in the IoT network. In 2015, Mishra et al. [22] suggested a password-based authentication scheme. That was resilient against some known security attacks. Both active and passive attacks can be resisted in addition to maintaining user secrecy. Additionally, it handles the user and gateway's mutual authentication. However, its operational cost is quite high along with the high overhead cost for gateway nodes. Hence, in reality, it becomes impracticable to implement.

Moon et al. [23] 2017 provided an effective password authentication for remote users. Their technique was based on smart card technology. The scheme enhanced the performance and security features but was unable to cater to user anonymity. Further, it did not provide security resistance against hidden gateway node attacks, spoofing attacks, or impersonation attacks. In 2019, Fatty and Amin [27] proposed an ElGamal cryptosystem-based scheme to provide security against all types of active and passive attacks. It has comparatively less computational cost compared to other schemes. In 2020, Vijaykumar P et al. proposed an authentication scheme having location privacy for IoT networks. The proposed scheme overcame the limitations of other schemes and provides authentication at a much lower computational cost [32].

Bera et al. [4] in 2020 recommended biometric based authentication schemes for the IoT application of smart cities by permitting a user that was registered with the network to renew their password using biometric authentication. The scheme is quite robust and is secured against all potential active and passive attacks. A biometric-based authentication strategy for smart cities for a worldwide mobility network was also proposed by Ghahramani et al. [9] (GLOMONET). While utilizing a single key, the system is effective and requires less communication. There was a about 53% reduction in the time complexity. By increasing the effectiveness of resources used in a variety of applications, including transportation, healthcare, and energy, Xie et al. [34] proposed a secure authentication strategy for the Internet of Things networks in the smart city. The efficiency of the system was demonstrated via formal verification based on pi calculations. A technique for authentication was also put up for smart cities by Xia et al. [33] to ensure improved data security and privacy. They demonstrated that this scheme is secured under the q-SDM problem and provides much better performance.

Table 6.1 displays the associated work's computation costs, communication costs, and other obstacles linked to cryptographic processes. The computational cost of the various secured authentication systems is shown in Fig. 6.3. Where indicated by the following

T_E – Time for exponential computation
T_H - Time for hash
T_M – Time for multiplication and division

Table 6.2 displays the suggested scheme's effectiveness in terms of time efficiency and energy consumption. According to the data in Xu et al. [35], for instance, the hash function TH requires 0.004 ms of execution time, the exponential function TE requires 0.16 ms, and the multiplication function TM requires 0.21 ms. These

Table 6.1 Comparison of computational costs, communication expenses, and security threats in different authentication schemes

Authentication scheme	Communication cost	Computational cost	Challenges of the schemes
Zhou et al. [37]	6 messages	$3T_{EM} + T_I + T_H$	False report injection, impersonation attack, denial of service, anonymity, gateway spoofing attack, forward secrecy, sensor spoofing attack, no mutual authentication
Huang et al. [10]	5 messages	$2T_{EM} + 5TH$	Sybil attack, impersonation attack, password guessing attack, no mutual authentication, anonymity attack
Huang et al. [11]	4 messages	$5TH$	User anonymity, Sybil attack, password guessing attack, untraceability, spoofing attack, no mutual authentication
Lee et al. [19]	5 messages	$2T_{EM} + 5TH$	Impersonation attack, password guessing attack, untraceability, spoofing attack, no mutual authentication, session key attack
Kim et al. [16]	4 messages	$2T_{EM} + 8TH$	Impersonation attack, denial of service attack, privilege attack, insider attack, untraceability, no mutual authentication
Huang et al. [12]	5 messages	$2T_{EM} + 2T_H$	Denial of service attack, privilege attack, insider attack, untraceability, spoofing attack, no mutual authentication, session key attack
Lee et al. [19]	4 messages	$2T_{EM} + 5TH$	Wormhole attack, impersonation attack, spoofing attack, no mutual authentication, session key attack
Turkanovic et al. [31]	4 messages	$23TH + 8T_E$	Denial of service attack, privilege attack, insider attack, untraceability, session key security, no mutual authentication
Mishra et al. [22]	3 messages	$19TH + 3T_M$	Wormhole attack, privilege attack, password guessing attack, untraceability, spoofing attack, no mutual authentication
Moon et al. [23]	4 messages	$17TH + 2T_E + 6T_M$	Impersonation attack, anonymity, gateway spoofing attack, sensor spoofing attack, no mutual authentication
Fatty et al. [27]	5 messages	$16TH + 4T_E + 6T_M$	Password guessing attack, impersonation attack no mutual authentication
Vijaykumar et al. [32]	4 messages	$12TH + 4T_E + 5T_M$	Anonymity, impersonation attack, denial of service attack, no mutual authentication
Bera et al. [4]	3 messages	$26TH + 2T_E + 2T_M$	Password guessing attack, anonymity, no mutual authentication

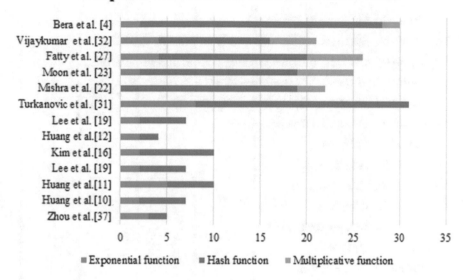

Fig. 6.3 Computational cost of various cryptographic secure access control schemes

Table 6.2 Time taken and energy consumption of various cryptographic schemes

Authentication scheme	Computational cost	Time taken	Energy consumption
Zhou et al. [37]	$3T_E + 2TH$	0.488	11.712
Huang et al. [10]	$2T_E + 5TH$	0.34	8.16
Huang et al. [11]	$5TE + 5TH$	0.82	19.68
Lee et al. [19]	$2T_E + 5TH$	0.34	8.16
Kim et al. [16]	$2T_E + 8TH$	0.352	8.448
Huang et al. [12]	$2T_E + 2\,T_H$	0.328	7.872
Lee et al. [19]	$2T_F + 5TH$	0.34	8.16
Turkanovic et al. [31]	$23TH + 8T_E$	0.7	16.8
Mishra et al. [22]	$19TH + 3T_M$	1.37	32.88
Moon et al. [23]	$17TH + 2T_E + 6T_M$	1.64	39.36
Fatty et al. [27]	$16TH + 4T_E + 6T_M$	1.96	47.04
Vijaykumar et al. [32]	$12TH + 4T_E + 5T_M$	1.73	41.52
Bera et al. [4]	$26TH + 2T_E + 2T_M$	0.844	20.256

values are computed in MI RACL using the C/C++ library. For the values of I = 8 mA and U = 3.0 V in active mode, we calculated the energy consumption using the formula E = U *I * t. The suggested design has undergone notable improvement, as seen in Table 6.2. Figure 6.4 shows the execution time and the energy consumption of the different authentication schemes.

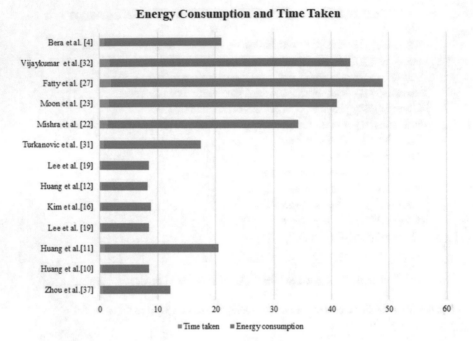

Fig. 6.4 Energy consumption and time taken of various cryptographic secure access control schemes

6.4   Conclusion

In this chapter, we've covered a variety of security requirements, as well as several security threats that could be present in IoT networks for digital medical records (DMRs). Then, some cryptographic systems have developed that address the flaws and provide strong security protections against a variety of active and passive assaults. We have also examined the computational costs and time complexity of several techniques that have been put out in the literature in this chapter. To determine the energy usage of various schemes, this study is beneficial. This paper provides a thorough overview of how to create an access control system that offers security protections with little computational and communication overhead.

References

1. Akyildiz, I., Su, W., Sankarasubramaniam, Y., & Cayirci, E. (2002). A survey on sensor networks. IEEE Communications Magazine, 76–88
2. Awoleye, O. M., Ojuloge, B., & Ilori. (2014). MO Web application vulnerability assessment and policy direction towards a secure smart government. Government Information Quarterly 31, 012, S118–S125. https://doi.org/10.1016/j.giq.2014.01

3. Batty, M., Axhausen, K. W., Giannotti, F., Pozdnoukhov, A., Bazzani, A., Wachowicz, M., Ouzounis, G., & Portugali, Y. (November 2012). Smart cities of the future. European Physical Journal Special Topics, 214(1), 481–518. https://doi.org/10.1140/epjst/e2012-01703-3

4. Bera, B., Das, A. K., Balzano, W., & Medaglia, C. M. (2020). On the design of biometric-based user authentication scheme in smart city environment. Pattern Recognition Letters, 138, 439–446, ISSN 0167-8655. https://doi.org/10.1016/j.patrec.2020.08.017

5. Burrows, M., Abadi, M., & Needham, R. (1990). A logic of authentication {J}. ACM Transactions on Computer Systems, 8(1), 18–36. https://doi.org/10.1145/77648.77649

6. Chan, H., Perrig, A., & Song, D. (2003). Randomkey predistribution schemes for sensor networks. In Proceedings of the IEEE Symposium on Security and Privacy (pp. 197–213), May 2003.

7. Choi, Younsung, Lee, D., Kim, J., Jung, J., & Won, D. Cryptanalysis of improved biometric-based user authentication scheme for C/S system. International Journal of Information and Education Technology, 5(7, July), 538–542. https://doi.org/10.7763/IJIET.2015.V5.564

8. Douceur, J. R. (2002). The Sybil attack. In. Lecture Notes in Computer Science. Proceedings of the 1st International Workshop on Peer-to-Peer Systems. IPTPS, 251–260. https://doi.org/10.1007/3-540-45748-8_24

9. Ghahramani, M., Javidan, R., & Shojafar, M. (2020). A secure biometric-based authentication scheme for global mobility networks in smart cities. Journal of Supercomputing, 76(11), 8729–8755. https://doi.org/10.1007/s11227-020-03160-x

10. Huang, H. F. (2009). A novel access control scheme for secure sensor networks. Computer Standards and Interfaces, 31(2), 272–276. https://doi.org/10.1016/j.csi.2008.05.014

11. Huang, H., & Liu, K. A new dynamic access control in Internet of things. (2008). IEEE Asia-Pacific services computing conference. https://doi.org/10.1109/APSCC.2008.116

12. Huang, H.-F. (2011). 'A New Design of Access control in Internet of Things' Hindawi Publishing Corporation. International Journal of Distributed Sensor Networks, 2011, article ID 412146.

13. Ilyas, M., & Mahgoub, I. (2005). Handbook of sensor networks: Compact wireless and wired sensing systems. CRC Press.

14. Karlof, C., & Wagner, D. (2003). Secure routing in Internet of things: Attacks and countermeasures IEEE International Workshop on Sensor Network Schemes and Applications (pp. 56–68).

15. Khaled, E. M., B. (2005). Drazen, C. Wang, and St Paul. Denial of service attack techniques: Analysis, implementation and comparison. Journal of Systemics, Cybernetics and Informatics, 3 – number 1, 66–71.

16. Kim, H. S., & Lee, S. W. (2009). Enhanced novel access control scheme over Internet of things. IEEE Transactions on Consumer Electronics, 55(2), 492–498. https://doi.org/10.1109/TCE.2009.5174412

17. Koblitz, N. (1987). Elliptic curve cryptosystems. Mathematics of Computation Math (Comp.), 48(177), 203–209. https://doi.org/10.1090/S0025-5718-1987-0866109-5

18. Lee, H., Shin, K., & Lee, D. (2009). Practical access control scheme for secure sensor. Networks 13th IEEE International Symposium on Consumer Electronics (ISCE2009).

19. Lee, H., Shin, K., & Lee, D. (2012). PACPs: Practical access control scheme for Internet of things 2012. IEEE Transactions on Consumer Electronics, 58(2), 491–499.

20. Malladi, Sreekanth, Alves-Foss, J., & Heckendorn, R. B. (2002). On preventing replay attacks on security schemes. Idaho University Moscow Department of Computer Science.

21. Miller, V. (1986). Uses of elliptic curves in cryptography, Advances in Cryptology-CPYPTO1985. Lecture Notes in Computer Science. Springer-Verlag, 218, 417–426.

22. Mishra, D., Das, A. K., Chaturvedi, A., & Mukhopadhyay, S. (2015). A secure password-based authentication and key agreement scheme using smart cards. Journal of Information Security and Applications, Appliance 2015, August 31, 23, 28–43. https://doi.org/10.1016/j.jisa.2015.06.003

23. Moon, J., Lee, D., & Jung, J. (2017). Improvement of efficient and secure smart card based password authentication scheme. IJ Netw. Security, 19(6), 1053–1061.

24. Mustafa, Y. H., & Hüseyin, A. (2013). Impersonation attack identification for secure communication. GLOBECOM Workshops, 1275–1279.
25. Nguyen, N. T., Reiher, P. L., & Kuenning, G. (2003). Detecting insider threats by monitoring system call activity. IEEE Workshop on Information Assurance (pp. 45–52).
26. R. Kirushnaamoni "Defenses to curb online password guessing attacks", Information communication and embedded systems (ICICES), 2013 international conference. (February 21 2013). On. IEEE Publications, 317–322.
27. Salem, F. M., & Amin, R. (2020). A privacy-preserving RFID authentication scheme based on El-Gamal cryptosystem for secure TMIS. Information Sciences, 527, 382–393. https://doi.org/10.1016/j.ins.2019.07.029
28. Shamir, A. (1979). How to share a secret. Communications of the ACM, 22(11), 612–613. https://doi.org/10.1145/359168.359176
29. Shen, J. et al. (2010). Comment: "enhanced novel access control scheme over Internet of things". IEEE Transactions on Consumer Electronics, 56(3), 2019–2021.
30. Tan, L., & Wang, N. (2010). Future Internet: The Internet of things. In ICACTE (Ed.). Proceedings of the 3rd International Conference Advance Compute. Theory Eng, 5 (pp. V5–V376)–V5-380, Aug..
31. Turkanović, M., Brumen, B., & Hölbl, M. (September 2014). A novel user authentication and key agreement scheme for heterogeneous ad hoc wireless sensor networks, based on the Internet of Things notion. Ad Hoc Networks, 20, 96–112. https://doi.org/10.1016/j.adhoc.2014.03.009
32. Vijayakumar, P., Obaidat, M. S., Azees, M., Islam, S. H., & Kumar, N. (April 2020). Efficient and secure anonymous authentication with location privacy for IoT-based WBANs. In IEEE Transactions on Industrial Informatics, 16(4), 2603–2611. https://doi.org/10.1109/TII.2019.2925071
33. Xia, X., Ji, S., Vijayakumar, P., Shen, J., & Rodrigues, J. J. P. C. (2021). An efficient anonymous authentication and key agreement scheme with privacy-preserving for smart cities. International Journal of Distributed Sensor Networks, 17(6). https://doi.org/10.1177/15501477211026804
34. Xie, Q., Li, K., Tan, X., Han, L., Tang, W., & Hu, B. (2021). A secure and privacy-preserving authentication scheme for wireless sensor networks in smart city. EURASIP Journal on Wireless Communications and Networking, 2021(1), 119. https://doi.org/10.1186/s13638-021-02000-7
35. Xu, L., & Wu, F. (2015). Cryptanalysis and improvement of a user authentication scheme preserving uniqueness and anonymity for connected health care. Journal of Medical Systems, 39(2), 10. https://doi.org/10.1007/s10916-014-0179-x
36. Yick, J., Mukherjee, B., & Ghosal, D. (2008). Wireless sensor network survey. Computer Networks, 52(12), 2292–2330. https://doi.org/10.1016/j.comnet.2008.04.002
37. Zhou, Y., Zhang, Y., & Fang, Y. (2007). Access control in Internet of Things. Ad Hoc Networks, 5(1), 3–13. https://doi.org/10.1016/j.adhoc.2006.05.014

Chapter 7
Integration of IoMT and Blockchain in Smart Healthcare System

7.1 Introduction

The network of hardware platforms, software programmes, and medical equipment that are all connected to the Internet for medical purposes is known as the Internet of Medical Things (IoMT). IoMT, also known as IoT in healthcare, enables wireless and remote devices to safely connect via the Internet to enable quick and adaptable analysis of medical data. The market for healthcare will unquestionably and permanently be affected by IoMT. A recent Deloitte survey predicts that the global IoMT market would increase from $41 billion in 2017 to $158 billion by 2022. The broader term for this is the Internet of Things (IoT), which refers to the network of all Internet-linked devices, such as connected factory equipment, biometric cyber-security scanners, and autonomous farming equipment. Healthcare and medical applications are the only focus of IoMT [1, 2]. With in-home IoMT, patients can send medical information from their residence to a hospital or their primary care physician. For instance, remote patient monitoring (RPM) [3] involves the use of medical devices to send data from recently discharged patients to their hospital for assessment by their doctors, such as blood pressure or oxygen saturation. By identifying problems early on, this can decrease hospital readmissions (Fig. 7.1).

Furthering patient flexibility, health – the use of communication technologies for remote healthcare services – allows freshly released patients to handle small concerns by remotely communicating with their doctors. For continued care away from the patient setting, IoMT devices combined with telehealth can be helpful. Personal emergency response systems (PERS) [4], for instance, can keep track of incidents like falls or heart attacks and instantly contact for assistance in those cases. At-risk individuals, such elderly who wish to live at home but are concerned about their safety, can find security with PERS. The internet of medical things is an application of the IoT for medical and health related purposes. Why do we need the IOT in healthcare? The answer to this question is the ageing of society, ageing of society

© The Author(s), under exclusive license to Springer Nature Switzerland AG 2023
S. Gupta et al., *Blockchain for Secure Healthcare Using Internet of Medical Things (IoMT)*, https://doi.org/10.1007/978-3-031-18896-1_7

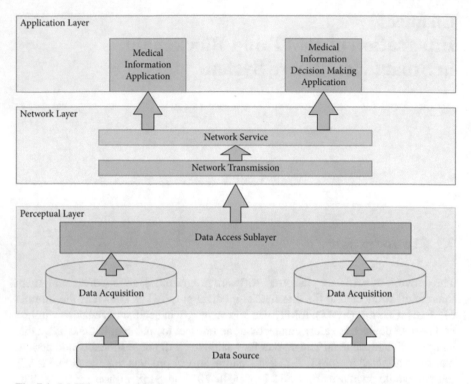

Fig. 7.1 IoMT layered architecture

means our society is gradually developing so we have to develop our healthcare systems also. As we can compare our current health system with the previous one, there is a big difference. Another reason we need IoMT is the shortage of medical staff. Especially in countries like India there is even unavailability of doctors so we should take the help of technologies. The other factor is diseases associated with wealth. With the help of the Internet of Things, it is possible to create a centralised network of connected objects that can produce and share data within a unified framework. IOT links hospitals and patients in this way. The ability to track and collect all of that data in real time results in the passive build-up of analytics data. Additionally, real-time information is tracked and gathered to enable quick response in an emergency. This implies that a standard hospital can be upgraded to a smart hospital in terms of improving medical facilities. Without a doubt, IoT is revolutionising the healthcare sector by changing how devices and people interact while providing healthcare solutions. IoT has applications in healthcare that benefit patients, families, physicians, hospitals and insurance companies. IoT can be used in many fields of area but its contribution in healthcare is great. In the current pandemic situation many IoT based wearable devices were used to check the signs of COVID-19 patients also for checking the oxygen percentage of every individual [5–7].

7.2   Benefits of IoMT in Smart Healthcare

Let us see now. Cost savings, better patient care, quicker illness diagnosis, proactive treatment, drug and equipment management, and less mistake are some benefits of IoMT in healthcare. So let's talk about all of IoMT's benefits for healthcare.

7.2.1   Cost Reduction

As we all know how much it costs in treatment as well as monitoring of patients in hospital. So IoT enables real time monitoring of patients. So it will reduce the cost of i = unnecessary visits to the doctor, hospital stay and readmission.

7.2.2   Improve Treatment

It enables physicians to make evidence-based informed decisions and brings absolute transparency.

7.2.3   Faster Disease Diagnosis

Real-time data and ongoing patient monitoring aid in early disease diagnosis – sometimes even before symptoms of the disease appear. Example: One of the most popular and crucial instruments for heart disease diagnostics is the ECG (Electrocardiogram). With the aid of this equipment, a doctor can evaluate a patient's heart rhythm, blood flow, tissue health, size, and anomalies by creating a visual representation of the heart's pulses. It is now possible to suit a patient with a portable ECG machine that can measure and record EKG readings anytime and anywhere utilising an IoT-based ECG monitoring system thanks to advancements in mobile and IoT technology [6, 7].

7.2.4   Drug and Equipment Management

More effective drug management is one of the Internet of Things' health advantages. The amount of medicine taken can be controlled thanks to IoT technology. Doctors can track therapy effectiveness and dose compliance. The Internet of Things also enables the ability to remind patients when it is time to take their medication.

When a patient doesn't take their medication on time, there are various circumstances in which the family member can be informed. In the healthcare sector, managing medications and medical equipment is a significant concern. These are efficiently handled and used at lower costs thanks to connected devices.

7.2.5   Error Reduction

In addition to assisting in better decision-making, data from IoT devices also helps to maintain smooth healthcare operations with decreased errors, waste, and system expenses. Many people pass away from chronic illnesses like heart disease, diabetes, and others. Patients may receive more individualised types of treatment and care because to the IoT's analytical capabilities. Elderly or patients with chronic ailments can have their health conditions monitored by smart, connected, or wearable devices [8]. With all of that information, medical professionals will be better equipped to treat patients and identify early disease indicators.

7.3   Tools and Technique for IoMT in Smart Healthcare

Smart healthcare is a health service system that uses technology such as wearable devices, IoT, and mobile internet to dynamically access information, connect people, materials and institutions related to healthcare, and then actively manages and afterward effectively oversees and reacts to clinical environment needs in a clever way. Smart medical services aren't a basic innovative progression, yet in addition an overall, staggered change. It comprises of numerous members, like specialists and patients, emergency clinics, and exploration organizations. It is an organic whole that includes numerous aspects, including infection anticipation and checking, determination and therapy, emergency clinic the board, wellbeing navigation, and clinical exploration. Data innovations, for instance, IoT, versatile Internet, distributed computing, large information, 5G, microelectronics, and computerized reasoning, along with current biotechnology establish the foundation of shrewd medical services. These advances are generally utilized in all parts of smart healthcare. According to the point of view of patients, they can utilize wearable gadgets to screen their wellbeing consistently, look for clinical help through menial helpers, and utilize remote homes to execute remote administrations. According to the viewpoint of specialists, an assortment of canny clinical choice emotionally supportive networks is utilized to help and further develop determination. Specialists can oversee clinical data through a coordinated data stage.

7.3.1   Electronic Health Record (EHR)

An electronic wellbeing record (EHR) framework gathers advanced wellbeing data for patients and the bigger populace. Different names utilized for this apparatus incorporate Electronic Medical Record (EMR) and Patient Health Record (PHR). Basically, it is a computerized adaptation of a patient's clinical history. The essential wellbeing supplier typically keeps up with the EHR. A patient's electronic wellbeing records might incorporate regulatory and clinical information like socioeconomics, meds, sensitivities, and clinical protection cover.

7.3.2   Referral Trackers

A reference global positioning framework is a product apparatus that medical care suppliers use to screen their patient references. It gives a successful correspondence channel between two clinical organizations. It additionally helps specialists and experts to keep up with consistent correspondence while dealing with a patient.

A reference apparatus empowers doctors to take care of numerous common-sense issues related with clinical references. For example:

- Doctors can utilize it to know the specific time their patient sees a subject matter expert and the consequence of the arrangement
- It disposes of the requirement for faxing reference letters
- It permits doctors to speak with a trained professional and choose if a patient's visit will be fundamental and helpful to the patient

7.3.3   Patient Portals

The Medlineplus.gov site characterizes a patient gateway as a site intended for your own medical care. It is an internet-based apparatus that empowers patients to screen their visits to their medical care supplier, check test results, charging, instillments, and solutions. A few gateways likewise permit patients to have live associations with their doctors and book new arrangements.

7.3.4   Remote Patient Monitoring

Distant patient checking (RPM) utilizes tech apparatuses to track and react to a persistent stream of patient information outside a medical clinic or center. This kind of telehealth is helpful for observing patients with ongoing conditions like cardiovascular breakdown, diabetes, and hypertension. Clinicians might utilize it to react instantly with a rescue vehicle when a patient's wellbeing information shows they are in critical need of crisis care.

7.3.5   Computerized Provider Order Entry

Automated supplier request passage (CPOE) frameworks should supplant the customary paper-based requesting framework. They permit clinicians to compose, send, and oversee different treatment directions, for example, lab tests, radiology orders, and prescription solicitations. Every one of these are done through a CPOE framework rather than through fax, printed paper, or phone.

7.4   Use Case of IoMT in Healthcare Industry

IoT has really many benefits but now lets see how the internet of things helps.

7.4.1   Internet of Things for Patients

Previously there was always a need of a medical person near you for checkups or for knowing your health conditions there was a need for checkups, but devices of IoT like fitness bands and other wearable devices which are also wireless which can also monitor blood pressure, heart rate (glucometer is used to measure the level of glucose in blood). These devices help the patients to take good care of their health. Also taking personal attention becomes easy by using these devices. There are also devices which show calories count, appointments, blood pressure variations and much more. A trustworthy heart activity tracker might be useful for fitness enthusiasts who keep tabs on their physical development. Users who occasionally have symptoms like irregular or skipped heartbeats but have not yet received a diagnosis for heart conditions such atrial fibrillation or AFib [9, 10]. They can keep track of and document these symptoms using the ECG app so that doctors can examine them further. Patients who already have heart conditions can track their well-being and recovery. IoT benefits patients and their families in this way.

7.4.2   Internet of Things for Hospitals

There are numerous other applications for IoT devices in hospitals besides patient health monitoring. The real-time position of medical equipment like wheelchairs, defibrillators, nebulizers, oxygen pumps, and other monitoring equipment is tracked using IoT devices tagged with sensors. Real-time analysis can also be done of the placement of medical personnel at various sites. Patients in hospitals are extremely concerned about the spread of infections. Patient infection can be avoided with the aid of IoT-enabled hygiene monitoring equipment. IoT devices are also useful for asset management tasks like controlling pharmacy inventory and checking refrigerator temperatures as well as controlling humidity and temperature in the environment. Also the ambulance of the hospital should have Remote ECG, BP sensors, 4G connectivity, Video uplink, communication links which will help in contacting hospitals and also monitoring the patient inside the ambulance [11].

7.4.3   Internet of Things for Physicians

Physicians can better monitor patients' health by utilising wearables and other home monitoring devices that are IoT-enabled. They can monitor a patient's adherence to their treatment regimen or any urgent medical needs. Healthcare personnel may now actively engage with patients and be more vigilant thanks to IoT.

7.4.4   Internet of Things for Business

IoT is bringing more business opportunities for the people as for storing large amounts of data and information we need a place in the cloud. So it provides valuable business advice for the outcome.

7.4.5   Internet of Things for Health Insurance Companies

IoT-empowered gadgets get a pool of chances to wellbeing safety net providers. Insurance agencies can utilise a lot of information gathered through various wellbeing observing gadgets for guarantee activities and endorsing. This will assist them with tracking down possibilities for guaranteeing and stay away from any sorts of phoney cases. The presentation of IoT gadgets in this area will get straightforwardness between the clients and guarantors as far as hazard appraisal processes, evaluating, guaranteeing, and asserts dealing with. The clients will actually want to have an unmistakable thought with respect to each choice taken and about its result as here activity cycles will be chosen in view of the information gathered from IoT-gadgets [12].

7.5 Privacy and Security Issue in IoMT

Telemedicine is a general term that covers all of the habits where you and your wellbeing supplier can use advancement to give without being in a comparative room. It fuses calls, video visits, messages, and texts. People similarly call it tele-health, modernized prescription, e-prosperity, or m-prosperity. There has been a many overlaps expansion in the reception because of COVID 19 and patients being not able to make a trip to meet specialists. It is vital to comprehend that telehealth is vulnerable to digital breaks and represents a monstrous danger to the classification, respectability, and accessibility of patients' electronic clinical records. Patient's clinical records contain exceptionally delicate data that ought not be made open to unapproved people to ensure patient protection, respectability, and privacy. The flip-side is that this data should be effectively accessible at whatever point needed by approved clients for a true reason. Telehealth presents all of the security issues as some other electronic transmission however, presumably perhaps the main issue will be accessibility – signal impedance, interference of transmission, or blackouts causing a main problem.

7.5.1 Patients Are Not in Charge of Their Own Information

IoMT and associated gadgets are pervasive in medical care as a result of the capacity to screen a patient's wellbeing progressively. Albeit these gadgets are vital to protecting numerous patients, it's vital to get the information that these gadgets are communicating. These gadgets and sensors can see when the patient is home, get communications with family, or distinguish different exercises the patient is partaking in, which may all be data the patient would prefer to keep hidden. The information gathered from these clinical gadgets can be put away by the gadget or application producer, in addition to the medical services supplier. This information could then be offered to outsiders and utilized for designated publicizing or even clinical mis-representation. Despite the fact that patients give agree to this assortment and capacity of information, security arrangements are frequently not perused or perceived by patients prior to concurring, considering more vulnerable protection insurances.

7.5.2 Present to Your Own Device (BYOD)

BYOD is when associations permit their representatives to involve individual gadgets for work purposes. Albeit these gadgets just access medical care frameworks and patient records through a VPN, that by itself isn't to the point of keeping endpoints secure. Forbes states that BYOD reception is speeding up in medical care likely because of medical care experts and suppliers who are presently telecommuting including clinicians, authoritative groups, monetary groups, and IT divisions. These experts are utilizing a wide cluster of gadgets like tablets, PCs, and phones for patient correspondence and different other work necessities, which builds the danger of information breaks. Medical services experts should be hyper watchful to guarantee no PHI is saved money on gadgets and that every gadget can be cleaned off somewhat on the off chance that it is taken or lost. Since the gadget, application, or program may not have a place with the supplier straightforwardly, safety efforts are difficult to monitor. There may likewise be a postponement of safety refreshes, unreliable associations or an absence of straightforwardness openly networks that could make wellbeing frameworks vulnerable to assaults.

7.5.3   Telecommuting Presents Security Chances

Representatives and project workers are additionally getting to the organization from a distance while telecommuting. The more individuals that are getting to the organization, the harder it is to monitor all clients and be aware of a deceitful or unapproved client. To remain as secure as could really be expected, it's vital to remember these telecommuting security tips.

7.6   Challenges of IoMT in Smart Healthcare

When there is opportunity, revolution then there are challenges too. So the internet of medical things (IoMT) has major challenges.

7.6.1   Underdeveloped Initiatives

IoMT devices are still growing and developing for battling chronic diseases. There are less organisations as well as people who are taking initiatives in developing and using internet of medical things devices.

7.6.2   Unavailability of Memory

As we know that we use IoT devices to keep monitoring the patients along with gathering and storing of their real time memory, so on using IoT devices and sensors there is a lot of data which we need to analyse so storing that much data is quite challenging due to lack of memory available.

7.6.3 Keeping Updated

We use many hardware as well as softwares in using IoT, so all the software should be regularly updated so that all the real time information can be analysed without any delay and the system runs smoothly.

7.6.4 Data Security

IoT is a system (hardware system) which works on the internet so hacking or manipulating of sensitive data is possible. The online system can be hacked so this can be a great challenge because all our private information can be manipulated or used for other unethical means [12, 13].

7.6.5 Global Healthcare Regulations

The Internet of Medical Things (IoMT) are still to be approved by the global health system. So approving the internet of medical things will take time. This is also restricting humans to innovate and use the internet of medical things [14, 15].

7.6.6 Scalable Platforms

Using IoT devices is also a challenge, as patients and doctors must be able to use the devices and also must be able to solve the technical issues. This requires an IoT platform which is user friendly, easy to use and scalable so that everyone can adapt it.

7.6.7 Data Overloading

We have earlier seen the data related issue, which was security but that is not only the challenge in internet of things and healthcare. As we know, IoT devices store more data and information and doctors have to analyse it so it is a huge problem for doctors to come to a conclusion. As more devices increase, data also increases and analysing them is more difficult [16].

7.7   Impact of IoMT on the Future of the Healthcare Industry

Telemedicine, also referred as e-medicine is defined as the use of telecommunications infrastructure and electronic software to consult, monitor and treat patients without the need for an in-person visit.

Telemedicine is an overall term that covers every one of the manners in which you and your health provider can utilize innovation to impart without being in a similar room. It incorporates calls, video visits, messages, and instant messages. Individuals likewise call it telehealth, computerized medication, e-wellbeing, or m-wellbeing. The computerized transmission of clinical imaging, far off clinical finding and assessments, and video meetings with experts are generally examples of telemedicine. A pre-set alarm can be sent to multiple groups using AI in a crisis situation, which will aid in saving a daily existence by making quick decisions. Therefore, with AI, medical professionals may easily manage patient records and provide after-hours medical services. Blockchain technology can also be used to provide security for an IoMT network. A distributed data set maintains secure, decentralised data electronically in a computerised architecture, ensuring the information's security and dedication. As a result, trust is built without the involvement of an outsider. Blockchain can be applied to the Internet of Medical Things (IoMT) [17] to provide security in medical servers that house electronic health records like MedRec, which can be used to manage access to and obtain approval for the sharing of medical information. We are then encouraged to conduct a close examination of various exploration issues examined by various specialists while developing an IoMT-based SHS. We are advised to work toward an artificial intelligence-based smart healthcare framework utilising the IoMT structure, taking into account the awareness of the current medical atmosphere. To assist adapt to the social distancing measures set up to assist with evening everything out of COVID-19 contaminations [18], the medical care industry needed to adjust rapidly. Telehealth turned into a redeeming quality for emergency clinics, facilities and specialists at the tallness of the pandemic looking for a method for giving a similar nature of care administrations while limiting the spread of the Covid. Key patterns have arisen encompassing the utilization of the innovation that will continue to shape the future of telemedicine services. Prior to the pandemic, telehealth administrations were for the most part restricted adhoc administrations with a huge scope of restrictions. Originally, they were made to help country and underserved patients get sufficiently close to experts when neighbourhood help was seriously limited. Jump forward to 2020–2021, and telehealth is becoming boundless across all parts of the business.

There is the prediction of number of changes:

- With a legitimate turn of events, wearables will tremendously affect medical services socially (improving the nature of patient consideration), financially (reducing down the expenses), and logically (empowering expansive resident science). Along with an adaptable plan of action and further developed information security, it is very equipped for making an upheaval around here.

- With the coming of more refined medical care IoT sensors and following instruments, the focal point of wellbeing wearables will move from customised wellness gadgets that rule the market these days to the clinical area's aggregate requirements.
- Inferable from the advancement of the Internet of Things and medical care, just as portable advances and Electronic Medical Reports (ERM), a gigantic measure of information will be produced. This reality will require the right and trustworthy handling of the wellbeing data and the arrangement of intuitive stages, bringing about new adaptation techniques.
- In the long haul, IoT advancement will bring a better way of life, decrease medical issues, the event of illnesses, and increment the productivity and accommodation of clinical benefits.

7.8　Conclusion

The medical care sector is experiencing extreme depression. The expense of health care administrations is higher than it has ever been, the global population is ageing, and the prevalence of chronic diseases is rising. A future that is rapidly approaching is one in which the vast majority of people would lack access to basic medical care, a significant portion of society would become useless due to advancing age, and people would be more susceptible to chronic sickness. Innovation can essentially simplify medical services by providing the patients with pocket-friendly clinical offices, even though it can't stop the population from ageing or instantly eradicate chronic illnesses. The Internet of Things (IoT) is a different viewpoint that has widespread martialness in many fields, including medicine. Utilizing this innovation-based medical services strategy has unmatched benefits that might improve the efficacy and quality of therapies and effectively improve the wellbeing of elderly patients.

References

1. Krishna, M & Neelima, M & Mane, Harshali & Matcha, Venu. (2018). Image identification using neural networks. 7. 614. https://doi.org/10.14419/ijet.v7i2.7.10892.
2. Huang, G.-B., Zhu, Q.-Y. & Siew, C.-K. Extreme learning machine: Theory and applications. Neurocomputing 70, 489–501 (2006).
3. Nguyen, G. et al. ML and DL frameworks and libraries for substantial and ample data mining: A survey. Artif. Intell. Rev. 52, 77–124 (2019).
4. Kshitiz, K., et al. "Detecting hate speech and insults on social commentary using NLP and machine learning." International Journal of Engineering Technology Science and Research 4.12 (2017): 279–285.

5. Hitesh Kumar Sharma; Anuj Kumar; Sangeeta Pant; Mangey Ram, "4 Application of Artificial Intelligence in Smart Healthcare," in Artificial Intelligence, Blockchain and IoT for Smart Healthcare, River Publishers, 2022, pp. 37–46.

6. Hitesh Kumar Sharma; Anuj Kumar; Sangeeta Pant; Mangey Ram, "5 Application of IoT in Smart Healthcare," in Artificial Intelligence, Blockchain and IoT for Smart Healthcare, River Publishers, 2022, pp. 47–56.

7. Hitesh Kumar Sharma; Anuj Kumar; Sangeeta Pant; Mangey Ram, "6 Application of Blockchain in Smart Healthcare," in Artificial Intelligence, Blockchain and IoT for Smart Healthcare, River Publishers, 2022, pp. 57–66.

8. Hitesh Kumar Sharma; Anuj Kumar; Sangeeta Pant; Mangey Ram, "7 Security and Privacy challenge in Smart Healthcare and Telemedicine systems," in Artificial Intelligence, Blockchain and IoT for Smart Healthcare, River Publishers, 2022, pp. 67–76.

9. Hitesh Kumar Sharma; Anuj Kumar; Sangeeta Pant; Mangey Ram, "8 Electronic Healthcare Record (EHR) Storage using Blockchain for Smart Healthcare," in Artificial Intelligence, Blockchain and IoT for Smart Healthcare, River Publishers, 2022, pp. 77–84.

10. Hitesh Kumar Sharma; Anuj Kumar; Sangeeta Pant; Mangey Ram, "9 Methodologies for Improving the Quality of Service and Safety of Smart Healthcare," in Artificial Intelligence, Blockchain and IoT for Smart Healthcare, River Publishers, 2022, pp. 85–94.

11. Hitesh Kumar Sharma; Anuj Kumar; Sangeeta Pant; Mangey Ram, "10 Cloud Commuting Platform for Smart Healthcare and Telemedicine," in Artificial Intelligence, Blockchain and IoT for Smart Healthcare, River Publishers, 2022, pp. 95–104.

12. Hitesh Kumar Sharma; Anuj Kumar; Sangeeta Pant; Mangey Ram, "11 Smart Healthcare and Telemedicine Systems: Present and Future Applications," in Artificial Intelligence, Blockchain and IoT for Smart Healthcare, River Publishers, 2022, pp. 105–116.

13. S. Kumar, S. Dubey and P. Gupta, "Auto-selection and management of dynamic SGA parameters in RDBMS," 2015 2nd International Conference on Computing for Sustainable Global Development (INDIACom), 2015, pp. 1763–1768.

14. Jing Tian, Boglarka Varga, Erika Tatrai, Palya Fanni, Gabor Mark Somfai, William F. Smiddy, and Delia Cabrera DeBuc. Performance evaluation of automated segmentation software on optical coherence tomography volume data. Journal of biophotonics, 9(5):478–489, 2016.

15. Ronald Klein and Barbara EK Klein. The prevalence of age-related eye diseases and visual impairment in aging: Current estimates. Investigative ophthalmology & visual science, 54(14), 2013.

16. R. Biswas et al. "A Framework for Automated Database Tuning Using Dynamic SGA Parameters and Basic Operating System Utilities", Database Systems Journal vol. III, no. 4/2012.

17. Sharma, Hitesh KUMAR. "E-COCOMO: the extended cost constructive model for cleanroom software engineering." Database Systems Journal 4.4 (2013): 3–11.

18. M. A. Abadi, P. Barham, E. Brevdo, Z. Chen, C. Citro, for example, is one of the most well-known companies in the world. Using Tensorflow, we can do large-scale machine learning on heterogeneous distributed systems. preprint arXiv:160304467 arXiv:160304467 arXiv:160304467 arXiv:1603044 (2016).

Chapter 8
Integration of IoMT and Cloud Computing for DMR Collection and Storage

8.1 Introduction

An active, global network infrastructure is coupled to self-configuring, intelligent sensors (objects) that make up the Internet of Things (IoMT) prototype [1]. In the IoMT, "things" can range from mundane objects that do not communicate to technological equipment that do. The IoMT is a technology that is expanding quickly [2]. IoMT typically has performance, reliability, security, and privacy difficulties according to physical and tiny sensors with limited capacity and memory [3]. The real sensor network is what is controlled and monitored online [4]. Utilizing Internet Protocol, applications, large-scale general-purpose computing, sensor networks, and communication technologies, the IoMT offers intelligent sensors [5]. The IoT prototype comprises of a self-configuring, intelligent sensor that is connected to a live, global network infrastructure [1]. A "thing" in the IoMT can be anything from a dull device that does not communicate to one that does. The Internet can be made up of smart sensors, tree trunks, or even a drink [6]. IoMT Idea finds a significant number of tangible items connected to [5]. There are currently 9 billion devices connected to the Internet. By 2020, they will have increased significantly and will number 24 billion. A more sophisticated technology with limitless processing and storage capacity is cloud computing. Cloud computing is the development and integration of adaptable, worldwide processing resources. Cloud resources come in a wide variety. To cut down on labour costs for service maintenance, cloud computing makes it easier to use remote configurable computing resources. Different virtualized assets are dispersed over numerous systems and domains as part of cloud computing. is frequently utilized by IoMT services because of its versatility and scalability. Consequently, it is typical for the IoMT and cloud combination to evolve on a wide scale. Next, we require a cutting-edge IT prototype. The cloud and the Internet of Things (IoMT) are two supporting composite technologies in this case that will disrupt the Internet both now and in the future [1]. IoT, big data, and cloud

S. Gupta et al., *Blockchain for Secure Healthcare Using Internet of Medical Things (IoMT)*, https://doi.org/10.1007/978-3-031-18896-1_8

computing working together provide several opportunities for businesses to experience exponential growth. IoMT is the data source, big data is the analytical platform, and cloud computing is the location of storage, scale, and access rates, to put it simply.

8.1.1   Big Data Relation with Cloud Computing

A massive dataset gathered by a significant network-based system is known as big data. This data is processed and accessed via the cloud, often utilizing a software as a service (SaaS) paradigm. To present the data to users, AI and machine learning are used. Cloud infrastructure offers efficient storage, real-time processing, and massive, quick analyses of big data, thus the two are mutually beneficial. The key advantage of using cloud storage for big data is its scalability. Cloud storage is a pay-as-you-go service. In its simplest form, the cloud is a platform that gives users access to and processing power over massive volumes of data. Big data analysis has a lot of promise since without cloud computing, today's computers cannot or are unable to evaluate this volume of data. Large data also contributes to the growth of cloud computing because there would be little need for cloud-based solutions without big data. So huge data cloud computing services are actually available. The availability of services that can gather, store, and process big data is the only justification for gathering big data. In other words, one cannot live without the other. Your organization can become a successful data-driven leader by combining the two.

8.1.2   Relationship Between IoMT and Big Data

The Internet of Medical Things is a global network of devices that collect and transmit information among numerous industries and businesses. On the other hand, big data makes it possible to handle and analyse enormous amounts of data across various platforms and systems. However, the compatibility of big data and the Internet of Things suggests that the two technologies have a similar future course and have a single goal in common.

8.1.3   Big Data and the Internet of Medical Things

Understanding IoMT and big data as different issues will make it easier for you to comprehend how closely they are related. The IoMT is the source of the data that your business needs to extract for analysis. Big data analysis and relevant data extraction can produce the information you require. Big data is essential for utilizing IoMT capabilities to extract data because it not only analyses massive amounts of data in real time but also employs a range of storage methods to store information. Data collecting is another difference. For instance, big data gathers information on human behaviour to identify patterns and make predictions. The equipment itself in order to achieve optimum performance and provide maintenance predictions, on the other hand, produces IoT data. However, they collaborate. The IoT gathers instant analytics data to aid with real-time decision-making. Predictive analytics uses big data as a storage solution, enabling it to anticipate future problems and create solutions, supporting this functionality. Inputs are examined, hidden connections and unknown patterns are revealed, and new trends in datasets are revealed by combining IoT with big data. IoT and big data are symbiotic, which means that as IoT expands quickly; strain on traditional data storage will grow, spurring the development of more creative big data solutions. Companies must therefore update their technology and processes to keep up with this expanding demand. Big data and the Internet of Things ultimately have a common goal and rely on one another to achieve it by transforming the data into something beneficial for the business. For instance, you may integrate current IoT insights with long-term big data analytics to get a more complete picture of your company's overall performance over time. With the development of these technologies, some industries will gain. The usage of IoT and big data will be advantageous for sectors including the transportation, shipping, and automobile industries. Technology-derived insights and insights enhance the analytical process, make it quicker and easier, increase efficiency, save expenses, and enable forecasting and decision-making with more knowledge [7].

8.1.4 IoT and Cloud Computing

When it comes to technical services, IoT and cloud computing are frequently branded together, complement one another, and work together to deliver better IoT services overall. However, there are significant distinctions between them that make them both individually and collectively an efficient technical solution. Collaboration is facilitated via IoT cloud computing, which is also used to store IoT data. You can use the cloud as a centrally located server with computational capabilities whenever you need to. The Internet may be easily used to transport huge amounts of data produced by the IoT via cloud computing. Here, big data is also helpful. Systems that offer real-time control and data monitoring can be automated affordably thanks to the Internet of Things and cloud computing [8].

8.1.5 Benefits of Using Big Data, IoT and the Cloud

Why then do big data, IoT, and the cloud work so well together? Utilizing these two services in tandem has a variety of benefits, some of which are outlined below.

- Data scalability on devices: To fulfil the needs of large data hosting and analytics, cloud-based systems can be scaled up and down. For instance, to enhance server capacity and add more hardware resources as needed, you can increase the number of apps. The development of big data and data analytics is made possible by the cloud.
- Scalable infrastructure capacity: Large amounts of data can be stored using a combination of big data and cloud storage, which also enables scalable processing and improved real-time data analysis. As big data, IoT, and the cloud do not require any physical infrastructure, you can cut costs and concentrate on your improved analytical capabilities without having to worry about upkeep or support.
- Increasing the effectiveness of routine work: Large volumes of data are produced through IoT and big data, and the cloud offers a means of transport for that data.
- The widespread acceptance and distribution of apps: You can increase cooperation by making it simple to access huge data remotely from anywhere in the world and continue using your device while accessing the cloud. Improvements in evaluating and monitoring linked IoT devices' status. Many devices might overload the Internet connection, and smart devices must send data to a server for processing rather than to a central server. This enables you to operate at the "edge" of your process, receive information from many network nodes, respond rapidly to outages, and anticipate when failures might happen. By delivering regular updates and instantly alerting authorities to infrastructure breaches, combining the cloud with the IoT can also improve security.
- Economies of scale benefits: efficiently storing and managing big data and IoT in the cloud may maintain corporate value. The cloud has apps, computing power, and administration tools built in for resource management.

8.2   IoMT Needs to Be Integrated with Cloud Computing

More significantly, the Internet of Medical Things (IoT) is cloud computing because it is so widely used that it must be allowed to consume the volume of data, virtual resources, and storage that it is capable of producing and give advantages may result from the integration [9] of IoMT-based cloud architecture.

The Fig. 8.1 shows the architecture that combines different parts to create an intelligent network of interconnected pieces, including sensor technology, gateways, RFID, and other intelligent technologies [10]. Figure 8.2 shows a straightforward IoT cloud system. The perceptual layer of human-worn IoT devices and sensors is where raw data is acquired. The network layer accesses data from Internet gateways. At the edge-computing layer, data preparation and cleaning are carried out. On the cloud platform, additional analysis and forecasts were carried out utilizing a variety of machine learning techniques. The primary objective of the Internet of Things (IoT) is to improve and simplify human life, either by assisting people in

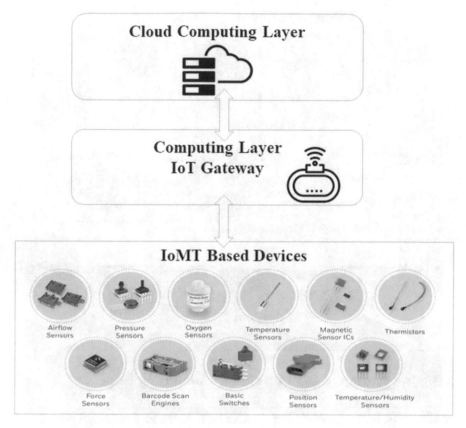

Fig. 8.1 IoMT based cloud architecture

making better decisions or by enabling them to live with less stress, repetitive work, and human contact.

Cloud computing requirements and implementations based on IoT applications for smart networks are tremendously in-demand right now across all industries. Agriculture, healthcare, education, smart cities, retail, and a number of other industries. IoT is utilised in agriculture to minimise transportation costs and pricing predictability based on historical data analytics [10]. IoT is frequently utilised in electricity conservation to inform consumers on electricity conservation [7] Numerous types of research are being conducted with the use of various IoT models in healthcare and various ways for disease prediction. When it comes to real-time patient health monitoring, IoT and cloud computing are highly useful. Sensor technology is employed, raw data is uploaded to the cloud for processing, and warning messages are given to the doctor and caregiver to interpret and forecast any illness or condition even in its early stages. For analysis and prediction, a variety of machine learning algorithms and data mining approaches are employed.

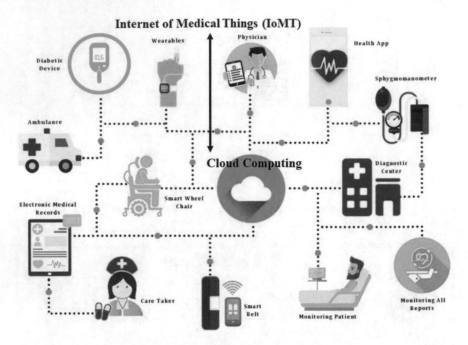

Fig. 8.2 Integration of IoMT and cloud computing

8.3 Integration of IoT and Cloud Computing

Additionally, a new generation of services built on the idea of "cloud computing" have evolved in recent years, reducing the need for hardware equipment and enabling access to information and data at any time, from any location. Or it was not included. The usage of computer software and hardware through the utilisation of services sent over the Internet is referred to as "cloud computing." The competition between large IT businesses and software is currently most intense in the area of cloud computing services [9]. When employing IoT, cloud computing can be employed as a foundational technology. Mobile cloud computing is more precisely described as the combination of cloud computing technologies and mobile devices, which results in mobile devices having abundant computation, memory, storage, power, and context-awareness resources. Increase. The consequence of an interdisciplinary strategy that blends mobile and cloud computing is mobile cloud computing [8]. Cloud computing additionally offers data processing, archiving, services, and applications via the Internet. An interdisciplinary approach that mixes mobile and cloud computing has led to the development of mobile cloud computing technologies. Therefore, mobile cloud computing is another name for this interdisciplinary field [7]. Storage over the internet, services over the internet, applications over the internet, and energy are a few of the fundamental aspects of cloud computing technologies that relate to the Internet of Objects characteristics of both things and effectiveness. IoT devices (such as mobile phones, sensors, and other IoT devices) can operate as interconnect systems for digital and personal information, which is a means for communities to live and interact. Key application areas that will profit from the development of IoT include smart grids and power systems, e-health and assisted living systems, industrial and environmental monitoring, and others. Globally, it is predicted that there will be 20 billion IoT-connected devices by 2023 [6]. Privacy concerns are growing as the number of IoT-enabled devices increases. Numerous sensitive data sets are produced, stored, and processed by such systems. It is becoming more challenging and complex to protect such data. With its abundant resources, cloud computing may be quite useful for managing and storing IoT data. IoT-based services can be successfully deployed in real time. Figure 8.2 illustrates the range of IoMT-based applications that can profit from cloud computing integration. Cloud computing, however, is susceptible to a range of harmful behaviors both inside and outside the cloud platform because it is thought of as a public and unprotected platform. As a result, successful integration of cloud computing and IoT-based applications requires a comprehensive data protection solution. In addition to developing an analytics service model that safeguards the privacy of cloud-based IoT applications, it is crucial to preserve the privacy of IoT data.

You have the chance to increase the utilization of deployed technologies in your cloud environment by combining the IoT and the cloud. Applications and data utilizing IoT technology will be accessible via cloud storage thanks to this connectivity. IoT and cloud technology integration, as depicted in Fig. 8.2.

8.4 Benefits of Integrating IoT and Cloud Computing

IoT and cloud systems working together offers several benefits. Here are some of the advantages explained. • Analysis – On the cloud platform, a sizable volume of unstructured sensor data is gathered.

- Cloud computing prototypes are used to capture aggregated sensor networks. You require more resources with this integration, study of this information, scalability (businesses can employ extra cloud vendor services for nothing), and integration. Scalability for sensor clouds refers to this. ## Visualization – Sensor's cloud infrastructure gives users a place to gather and be creative.
- Gather data on sensors from numerous sources.
- Coordination Integrate many physical sensor networks so that retailers across different categories can exchange sensor data via the sensor cloud
- Enhancements to data processing and storage – Allocation of superfluous processing and storage.
- Offering tools and programmes for handling massive amounts of data. • Sensor cloud with dynamic service processing allows data access from anywhere, at any time.
- Has convenient access to sensor data.

- Flexibility: Users are free to expand on earlier computation techniques. It benefits us
- Store and distribute sensor data in a range of settings. • Daisy Chain Wireless Sensor Networks (WSN) with Cloud Computing for Quick Response
- Quickly responding users. It is therefore regarded as a real-time application.
- Automation – In sensor cloud computing, automation is crucial. Additionally, it is rising when to submit significant amendments
- Multi-tenancy – This refers to the capability of distributing the service to numerous users and allowing them to share cloud resources.

8.5 Conclusion

Cloud computing technology has a lot of potential, but it also has significant restrictions. The term "cloud computing" describes an infrastructure where both data processing and storage take occur off mobile devices. An overview of Internet of Things technology, including how it functions and how to use it, is provided in this chapter. Additionally, it discusses the main advantages and disadvantages of cloud computing. The term "cloud computing" describes an infrastructure where both data processing and storage take occur off mobile devices. Another quickly developing new technology in the telecommunications industry, particularly in contemporary cellular telecommunications, is the Internet of Things. The main objective of interaction and collaboration between objects and objects sent across a wireless network is to achieve the goals established as a single organism. Additionally, because both cloud computing and Internet of Things depend on wireless network technologies, both fields are developing swiftly. This white paper provides an introduction of IoT and cloud computing with a focus on security issues related to each technology. We will explicitly integrate the two technologies (cloud computing and IoT) listed above to look at their similar traits and discover the benefits of their combination.

References

1. Alessio Botta, Walter de Donato, Valerio Persico, Antonio Pescapé, Integration of Cloud computing and Internet of Things: A survey, Future Generation Computer Systems, Volume 56, 2016, Pages 684–700, ISSN 0167-739X, https://doi.org/10.1016/j.future.2015.09.021
2. J. Gubbi, R. Buyya, S. Marusic, M. Palaniswami Internet of Things (IoT): A vision, architectural elements, and future directions Future Gener. Comput. Syst., 29 (7) (2013), pp. 1645–1660
3. Abdulatif Alabdulatif, Ibrahim Khalil, and Syed Hassan Ahmed, Integration of Internet of Things (IoT) and Cloud Computing: Privacy Concerns and Possible Solutions, IEEE Internet Policy Newsletter, September 2018
4. M. R. Rahimi et al, "Mobile Cloud Computing: A survey, State of Art and Future Directions", Mobile Networks and Applications, Volume 19, Issue 2, pp. 133–143, 01/04/2014.
5. Jiehan Zhou et al, «CloudThings: a Common Architecture for Integrating the Internet of Things with Cloud Computing», in Huazhong University of Science and Technology, Wuhan, 2013.

6. Chacko V and Bharati V 2017 IEEE International Conference on IoT (iThings) and IEEE GreenCom and IEEE CPSCom and IEEE SmartData, pp. 906–909.
7. Botta A., de Donato W., Persico V. et al.: 'Integration of cloud computing and internet of things: a survey', Future Gener. Comput. Syst., 2016, 56, pp. 684– 700.
8. Gubbi J., Buyya R., Marusic S. et al.: 'Internet of things (Iot): A vision, architectural elements, and future directions', Future Gener. Comput. Syst., 2013, 29, (7), pp. 1645– 1660.
9. Rajabion L., Shaltooki A.A., Taghikhah M. et al.: 'Healthcare big data processing mechanisms: the role of cloud computing', Int. J. Inf. Manage., 2019, 49, pp. 271– 289.
10. Khorshed M.T., Sharma N.A., Kumar K. et al.: 'Integrating internet-of-things with the power of cloud computing and the intelligence of big data analytics—A three layered approach'. 2015 2nd Asia-Pacific World Congress on Computer Science and Engineering (APWC on CSE), Nadi, Fiji, 2015

Chapter 9
Methodologies for Improving the Quality of Service and Safety of Smart Healthcare System

9.1 Introduction

The introduction of the IoT paves the way for the development of smart healthcare functions that mix the well-known and well-accepted digital applied sciences [1]. The IoT can help to interface such autonomous devices to communicate with each other without the involvement of humans and give characteristic data or results as an outcome [2]. Intelligence is needed to classify this inherent data and generate it in such a way that it is accessible to the individuals in the process of making decisions [3]. In the year 2011, the arena population reached 7 billion, and the variety of connected contraptions stood at 13 billion [4]. By the approach of 2016, there may be over three times the number of connected contraptions as people in the world, and 5 years later, there will probably be 50 billion connected devices for many effective seven. 6 billion individuals (Inspiring the Internet of Things, 2016) [5]. We are witnessing the comeback of the internet's customary style. The terrible idea of the internet was to connect various things. Recently, there are already several matters that confine bits with various things, but traditionally they need to be used protocols aside from the online protocol (IP) [6], and communication takes the state of affairs over temporary distances, for example, in electronic locks and key cards. What is new regarding IoT is that communication will take place in an impartial position [7].

The long-established web won't be regarding communications as a way of providing offerings [8]. The subsequent stage of this development may be a convergence of offerings with immensely shared information. It is not possible without a classy wireless and sticks infrastructure to allow access anywhere, whenever associated growing and present material links people and desktop-to-laptop communications [9].

© The Author(s), under exclusive license to Springer Nature Switzerland AG 2023
S. Gupta et al., *Blockchain for Secure Healthcare Using Internet of Medical Things (IoMT)*, https://doi.org/10.1007/978-3-031-18896-1_9

9.1.1   IoT in Smart Healthcare Systems

Traditional healthcare systems are experiencing numerous issues as the world's elderly population grows. Healthcare costs have risen due to an exponential increase in the number of elderly individuals in wealthy countries [10]. The growing elderly population has posed significant issues for policymakers, healthcare professionals, hospitals, insurance companies, and patients. One of the most difficult issues in providing improved healthcare to an expanding number of people is a lack of financial and human resources [11].

IoT refers to any physical object installed with innovation fit for trading information and is pegged to make a more productive healthcare framework regarding time [12], vitality, and cost. One zone where innovation could be demonstrated transformative is healthcare—with experts at MarketResearch.com asserting the area will be worth $117 million by 2020 [13].

By implanting IoT-empowered devices in restorative hardware, healthcare experts will have the capacity to screen patients all the more successfully—and utilize the information gathered from the devices to make sense of who needs the most hands-on consideration [14]. At the end of the day, by benefitting as much as possible from this system of devices, healthcare experts could utilize information to arrange proactive administration—as it's been said, avoidance is superior to the cure [15].

Connected prosperity remains the snoozing enormous of the web of issues applications. The motivation of a connected human services approach and keen clinical contraptions bears gigantic gifts [16], no longer just for organizations furthermore for the prosperity of individuals much of the time [17]. However, connected health has now not achieved the majority but rather. IoT in Healthcare is a heterogeneous registering, remote technique of applications and contraptions that associates patients and prosperity suppliers to analyze, screen, screen, and store critical data and therapeutic data [18].

An insightful healthcare strategy must provide care to people in far-flung areas and check programs that give consistent information to move for better decisions [19]. IoT changes a healthcare method by methods for significantly bettering incredible and IoT will achieve an astute medicinal services technique to people [20]. In this part, we depict diagrams of our plan for a canny healthcare technique called IOT Healthcare and the rightful design of IoT human services. Sagacious medicinal services assume a giant part in human services capacities through installing sensors and actuators in patients and their solutions for observing and checking purposes [21]. The IoT is used by logical care to watch the physiological statuses of sufferers using sensors as a method for gathering and breaking down their knowledge, after which dissecting the patient's data remotely to handling focuses to make appropriate activities. IoT can be used to supplement sufferers' cures through far-away checking and verbal trade and to keep up a screen of patients as they move using a medicinal services office. Read on to find the specifics of those IoT arrangements [22].

From associated ice chests that demonstrate the contemporary family unit pics to related catches that quickly area a request for clothing cleanser while you squeeze them [23], the Internet of Things is sizeable and growing quickly. Prosperity mind simply isn't impervious to this new connected fever. Health care pioneers and trend-setters are rapidly building up connected health things that present solid new strategies to deal with people [24].

Every time, associated health-connected science can give intense and perhaps lifesaving understanding, and in various circumstances, they may, with no inconvenience, outfit the extra inspiration needed to ascend and get moving [25]. Connected prosperity is influencing charming steps to sustain our capacity to seize, investigate, and eventually benefit from our prosperity data [26].

9.2   Background/Present State in Data Security

Active and passive attacks are the two broad classifications of security threats. The attacks that do not affect the resources of the system instead try to learn useful system information through passive attacks [27]. Moreover, system confidentiality is highly compromised by this kind of attack. Conversely, attacks affecting the normal operation of the system or altering the system resources are called "active attacks." On the hand, the availability or integrity of a system is compromised by this kind of attack. Unencrypted traffic is keenly monitored by a passive attack to make worthless the routing of sensible data to the desired destination [28].

In smart healthcare systems, the information could be shared securely in an effective way. This technology was allowed by computer networks. A network is fixed into two options: wired and wireless networks [29]. Wired networks have connected the computers with the support of networking cables. Conversely, wireless networks have connected computers using radio frequencies [30]. Recently, wired and wireless networks are highly adopted by most developing organizations. Common differences found between wired and wireless networks are one uses network cables and the other one uses the radio-frequencies for communication [31]. However, secure communication can be provided using a wired network only at 2000 feet shortest distance. Outside interference and high transmission speeds can make wireless networks less secure during communication. None of the computer networks is wholly safe or secure [32]. The techniques of data security in smart healthcare as shown in Fig. 9.1.

Individuals and organizations have considered preserving network security a great deal because of its vital role in information storage and processing the business using the internet. An organization will enter into trouble when security is compromised or with the sudden failure of the network [33]. The only safe way to improve communication using wireless networks is keeping away unauthorized users or attackers away from accessing the networks. Considerably, active and passive attacks are the two broad classifications of security threats [34]. The attacks that are not affecting the system resources but instead; trying to learn the useful

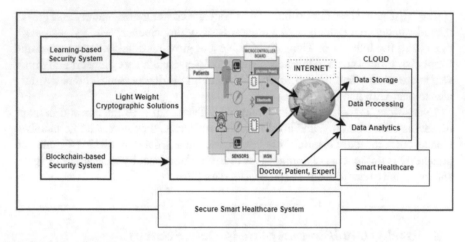

Fig. 9.1 Data security techniques in smart healthcare

system information is called passive attacks [35]. Moreover, system confidentiality is highly compromised by this kind of attack. Conversely, the attacks affecting the normal operation of the system or altering the system resources are called to be active attacks [36]. On the hand, the availability or integrity of a system is compromised by this kind of attack. Unencrypted traffic is keenly monitored by a passive attack to make worthless routing of sensible data to the desired destination [37].

Some of the illegal activities included in passive attacks are, capturing most authenticated data (i.e., passwords), decrypting poorly encrypted data, monitoring vulnerable communication, analyzing traffic, and so on. However, without requiring the knowledge of the user, the data files or sensitive information are disclosed by the passive attackers [38]. Breaking or bypassing the unauthorized system by an attacker is the main functionality of an active attack. Active attacks are highly supported when the management or operation violates the policies of system security, implementation, and system design that are exploited with the presence of Trojan horses, worms, viruses, and stealth. Some of the activities, such as data modification, denial of service, and dissemination or disclosure of data files, are the outputs of active attacks. A distributed attack is the most significant type of active attack.

A distributed attack mainly focuses on the trusted software or system to insert malicious code (such as a backdoor program or Trojan horse) by initiating an attacker. In too many vulnerable systems, the self-propagation or distribution of malicious code is done to generate a botnet (i.e., compromised hosts are connected to the created network of the internet). Using an external standard network protocol, the botnet containing compromised hosts is controlled remotely. Smart healthcare distributed attacks are launched using these compromised hosts, which in turn support malicious activities. Distributed Denial of Service (DDoS) attack is one of the most commonly known types of distributed attacks.

The income misfortune has enhanced to $209 million in 2016 when contrasted with $24 million for all of 2015 [39]. As per the ongoing Worldwide Infrastructure Security Report (WISR), the traffic volume of such assaults has enhanced to around 650 Gbps in the year 2016. It is clear from this exponential increment in assault traffic that the aggressors are continually refreshing their aptitudes, utilizing propelled systems to create such a gigantic measure of traffic and simultaneously crushing the current resistance arrangements. Some ongoing DDoS pattern reports found that the recurrence of DDoS assaults is up by 129% in the last quarter of 2016 contrasted and a similar period a year ago. It implies there is no sign to battle against such assaults successfully in the not-so-distant future as well.

9.2.1   Data Security Requirements in Smart Healthcare Systems

Five different data security requirement axes in smart healthcare systems are (a) availability; (b) authenticity; (c) confidentiality; (d) integrity; and (e) non-repudiation. One of the most complex issues to be faced is securing network communications in smart healthcare systems, which has numerous challenges [40].

- **Availability:** An availability issue to be known is maintaining the functionality of networks. Notably, the presence of communication bandwidth and the required service or information should be ensured by a security framework at any given time. In the infrastructure environment, cryptography and trust-based solutions have allowed network security. Also, in the case of fully distributed scenarios, the trust-based solution alone can provide a better option compared to cryptography-based approaches.
- **Authenticity:** Access control, authentication, and identification are the major security concerns to be considered during data transmission.
- **Confidentiality:** Confidential peer-to-peer communication can be made by encrypting all the exchanged messages, shared public keys, and certificates. Compared to trust-based solutions, cryptography-based solutions have ensured confidentiality.
- **Integrity:** To verify the status of transmitted messages, whether they have been reduced, modified, or dropped in an intermediate node, trustworthiness, and data integrity assurance has played a core role. In a distributed system, achieving this requirement is a complex task.
- **Non-repudiation:** Any node trying to forger any of the sent messages can be easily detected using cryptographic-based solutions.

Table 9.1 Various security attacks in Smart Healthcare Systems

Nature of attack	Description	Classification
Active attacks	These are performed mainly to carry out malicious acts against the system, thus affecting or disrupting the services for legitimate users. They hamper both the confidentiality and integrity of the system.	Dos (denial-of-service), DDOS (distributed denial of service), MITH (man-in-the-middle), Interruption, Alteration [47].
Passive attacks	These are performed mainly for gathering useful information without getting sensed, i.e., they do not disturb the communication.	Monitoring, traffic analysis, eavesdropping, node destruction/malfunction [49].
Privacy threats	The capabilities of IoT allow it to launch acute attacks targeting the privacy of users.	Identification, profiling, tracking, linkage, inventory
Protocol-based attacks	The attacks work against the connectivity protocols of IoT.	RFID-based (replay, tracking, killing tag) Bluetooth-based (bluesnarfing, bluejacking, Dos), Zigbee based (sniffing, replay, ZED sabotage attack)

9.3   Privacy and QoS in Smart Healthcare

- Despite promising prospects for IoT and its QoS in the smart healthcare sector, there are still hurdles and an express level of uncertainty that may confirm and shape how clinical care may benefit from this paradigm change in health supply [41]. Table 9.1 tabulated the various security attacks in Smart Healthcare Systems.

Some of the privacy issues and considerations of smart healthcare include,

- Reluctance or hesitation on the part of traditional aid providers to transfer to the current new method of business. We anticipate that, in time and due to the cost-effectiveness of smart healthcare systems, the majority of providers will seek to take advantage of the benefits afforded by deploying smart healthcare solutions in their network. Similarly, patients' aversion to interacting with and employing smart healthcare system-related technologies will be eliminated through education and awareness [42].
- Security and privacy concerns must be addressed before any IoT-based device can be fully enjoyed. Because knowledge collection, mining, and provisioning are done through the internet in such systems, unauthorized actors can invade. In brief, the flow of huge amounts of knowledge within the ever-expanding IoT applications, as well as the security issues that may still arise, necessitate extensive investigation in areas such as dynamic trust, security, and privacy management. Despite resource constraints in terms of energy convenience and procedural capabilities, new and inventive solutions are nevertheless required to provide an adequate level of security.
- Another challenge is the acquisition, management, and reliable analysis of huge amounts of information generated by the patient population's massive flow of

data. It is critical to streamline the automation and analysis of this vast knowledge and establish a suitable way of informing physicians and other stakeholders in an extremely timely manner. Furthermore, even though the value of storage is decreasing, we are still obligated to reduce the value of retaining this knowledge by building intelligent algorithms that will facilitate the removal of superfluous knowledge [43].

- The appearance of wearable sensors and power consumption continue to be issued in health-related IoT deployments. The subject of how to gain inconspicuousness while watching patients remains open because comfort, whereas observance, could be a fundamental goal. Patients may be burdened by the necessity for frequent recharging of reversible batteries [44]. As a result, reducing energy consumption could be a significant restriction. At the moment, alternatives such as energy harvesting and alternative energy area units are being researched, while research activities aimed at establishing communication protocols and sensors with low energy consumption area units are continuing [45].

9.4   Data Security and Privacy Issues in Healthcare

Data security refers to digital privacy safeguards that can be implemented to prevent unwanted access to computer systems, databases, and websites. Data protection also safeguards against data corruption. Information security is a top responsibility for businesses of all sizes and types. Information security is often referred to as know-how security or computer security.

IoT can provide data that is far superior to traditional analytics by utilizing devices that can perform capability research. As a result, IoT aids in healthcare by providing more realistic and reliable statistics, yielding higher answers, and the discovery of previously undisclosed difficulties, which is why studies are one of the most important IoT applications in healthcare [46].

Devices
Even though modern devices are improving in terms of strength, precision, and availability, they still offer fewer benefits and functionality than IoT devices. IoT has the potential to liberate the current generation and bring us closer to advanced healthcare and medical tool solutions.

IoT Hardware & Software in Depth
IoT attempts to bridge the gap between how we deliver healthcare and the device by designing a device rather than merely equipment. It then identifies problems, well-known styles, and missing features in healthcare.

Care
IoT enables healthcare providers to use their knowledge and education to tackle problems more effectively. It enables them to use superior data and technologies, which aid in extra-unique and swift motions during the flip. IoT allows healthcare

professionals to advance professionally by allowing them to spend less time on administrative tasks and more time practicing their skills.

IoT Applications in Media, Marketing, and Advertising
One of the most notable innovations of IoT applications in healthcare is the provision of correct and up-to-date records to patients, which remains one of the most difficult difficulties in medical treatment. IoT devices not only improve fitness in people's daily lives; but also in facilities and professional exercise.

IoT solutions move healthcare out of hospitals and allow for intrusive care in the workplace, home, or social setting. They empower and enable people to care for their health, allowing healthcare providers to provide better treatment to patients. As a result, fewer accidents have occurred as a result of a misunderstanding, improved patient satisfaction, and better preventive treatment.

Emergency Care
The emergency assistance options have consistently been plagued by limited sources and becoming detached from the base facility. IoT's sophisticated automation and analytics address this issue in the healthcare sector. An emergency can be assessed from a long distance, or even miles away. Companies have access to patient profiles far ahead of their arrival, allowing them to provide critical care to patients on time. As a result, related losses are decreased, and emergency health treatment is prioritized.

The IoT has a wide range of applications, one of which is social insurance. Sensors are either worn by the person or placed in the person's environment. These sensors collect data relating to a person's lifestyle and physiological and psychological well-being, and this data can be collected, saved, and analyzed to bring about a positive change in the person's life. This access to information would aid in appropriate diagnosis and foresee fatal complications, and if accompanied by counteractive action, the prospect of healing the condition and restoring health would be realized. This would also allow for customization of treatment and consideration of the patient's wants. This treasure trove of data may be collected and displayed to health care providers and doctors in a straightforward manner, reducing expenses. However, there were significant challenges with identification, analysis, and comprehension that needed to be addressed before deploying the framework on a large scale in a clinical context.

It has to be seen how cloud computing will affect the healthcare sector because it is very diverse, complicated, and unique and offers several challenging conditions, such as guarding people's health data in addition to adhering to HIPAA recommendations provided by federal compliance rules. The ever-increasing expense of healthcare solutions exacerbates these difficulties. Attempts are being made to minimize the fees that clients must pay and to provide better medical services, but this will take time.

IoT devices have various applications such as e-Health, online business, e-Home, e-Trafficking, etc. As so many applications are feasible, it raises security concerns and protection issues. There have been many studies conducted on security challenges in IoT, but the actual investigation of these challenges is absent.

In this book chapter, an extensive exploration of IoT security complications and issues has been done. IoT assault surfaces, risk models, security issues, necessities, legal sciences, and difficulties have been discussed in depth. The open issues in IoT security and protection have been addressed, and the basic issues are taken care of. Issues identified due to interoperability of different devices used in the IoT are also being investigated, and vulnerabilities have been presented based on factors such as computational restriction, vitality impediment, asset constraint, and lightweight cryptographic conventions. Also, the dangers of not having a proper IoT security procedure have been laid out.

9.5   QoS Parameters for Smart Healthcare

In smart healthcare, the QoS is considered the most challenging since the resources like sensors availability and several applications that run on the networks might have various constraints to meet the requirements. Quality of service could be measured at the network level regarding the delay, jitter, bandwidth limitation, and throughput.

Whereas accommodating security will construct trade-off options dynamically based on the threat state of affairs. However, there is insufficient evidence to show how such an answer might appear in an extremely heterogeneous and lightweight objects-driven network like the IoT, and to what extent it is possible. The goal is to create a context-aware adaption model that will associate a threat in a larger context to avoid false alarms and can modify security improvements autonomously by the user, QoS, and resource needs.

Few network design challenges that impact QoS are as follows [47].

- **Limited energy capacity**: The consumption of energy by hardware and software is the principal factor in the network. The handling of energy in an efficient manner prolongs the network lifetime.
- **Limited hardware resources**: The hardware like storage and its energy computation should be managed with constrained energy consumption along with the protocol design and its software development for communications.
- **Random deployment**: In most cases, sensor nodes are deployed either manually or randomly based on the requirements of the application. After the deployment, they should be capable of organizing themselves for further communications.
- **Unreliable and Dynamic environment**: Due to the disrupted network connectivity and frequent changes in the network topology, the nodes in the WSN operate in an unpredictable and dynamic environment.
- **Diverse applications**: The requirements of the sensor node are application-specific and the concern nodes are integrated according to the application requirements.

9.6   Suggested Security Techniques to Preserve QoS

With advancements in the areas of network and information security, network economics can be achieved, and this can be done using a technique called web data mining. This enhances the performance of data security in the network and primarily deals with the analysis of information security by making use of such data mining techniques. Considering the meta-analysis using the web data mining technique, it is feasible to achieve information security, and a web mining prevention model is used for the purpose to preserve QoS. The results can be accurate and valuable, and more priority is assigned to sensitive data. Scenarios where one can prevent hackers from getting access to such sensitive data.

Today, RFID advances are being connected to a smart sensor framework to enhance the nature of the social insurance framework. Security and protection issues in RFID frameworks and IoT-based applications. Remote sensor systems can be connected for universal health checking, enhancing clients' prosperity, making the human services framework more proficient, and serving to rapidly respond to crisis circumstances. Adhering to the strict security requirements of omnipresent restorative applications can become a major test. The authors also reviewed a sending model for unavoidable medical services concerning tolerant zone and therapeutic sensor systems.

IoT security improvements are essential for smart healthcare systems and to preserve QoS. A few issues and arrangements from each layer of the IoT security structure. Advanced security conventions and instruments are utilized for the elite and security in the medical services framework. Also, the security issues related to IoT development layers are examined, and suitable adapting systems are given to fabricate a safe IoT development so the IoT can ensure solid and stable advancement in reasonable applications. A test sooner rather than later will be the reconciliation of IoT with security conventions to the healing center condition. Building up a security convention in u-medical services condition is a real worry in the future.

IoT devices being utilized currently have implementations that keep their legitimate use in human services frameworks. Interoperability and security are particularly affected by such constraints. In this work, the authors present issues, including advantages and challenges, and, in addition, ways to deal with and overcome the issues of applying and incorporating IoT devices into human services frameworks. The REMOA project is considered a case study in which the focus is on an answer for homecare or tele-observing for patients with endless diseases.

The experiment reported on the exploitation of ready-to-wear IoT devices for telemonitoring reception of healthcare applications showed that though possible, the emerging market still doesn't supply a versatile product that will be simply tailored to be used in contexts except the offered by the manufacturer which permits solely access to servers that have been configured beforehand in some cases. Hence, it can be observed that there are problems that are still in the early stage and properly not investigated transfer system that connects the healthcare suppliers to the patients. This becomes a limitation when desegregation of IoT devices is done for a very broader setting. Service-Oriented Architectures (SOA) mechanisms are used by many middleware systems and act as a basis for a middleware design in embedded networks. But there is a necessity for enhanced standards of devices, particularly within service devices. Required criteria ought to cover open genus API's selection of interconnection interfaces, and configuration choices of the operational mode of the monitoring/control device, together with the aggregation of extra security mechanisms.

Presently the IoT devices that are used can easily be made to overcome limitations in medical healthcare applications, especially the Security & Interoperability issues. In this study, issues, challenges, advantages, and methodologies that have been developed for rectifying the issues and calibrating the IoT devices in the healthcare sector have been discussed. Also, the case study considered here is the REMOA project. This project deals with telemonitoring of chronically or terminally ill patients.

Readily available IoT gadgets that can be used in the implementation of tele monitoring applications can be realized but the industry is unable to cope and provide the devices that can seamlessly integrate and still the producer has to grant permission to be able to access the preconfigured servers as and when required. There are issues with IoT interoperability as information exchange between devices that are connected in the network have social insurance issues with suppliers and patients. If a more extensive setting is required, this becomes even more problematic. There are however a few middleware gadgets that use SOA for middleware design in embedded networks. Even so, the need for improving interoperability is a must, especially for applications that deal with the healthcare and medical sectors.

Open APIs, interfaces for interconnection, and several configuration options for operation modes of the monitoring/control device and additional security mechanisms have to be incorporated. This study proposes a solution to the interoperability issue by introducing an embedded middleware and setting up specific IoT devices for wireless health monitoring devices utilizing the Wi-Fi interfaces available. The downside is that such devices cannot be directly associated owing to security issues. However, it is always possible to involve an improved AAA (Authentication, Authorization, and Accounting) supplier for this purpose. One major advantage is that the no-cost product can have a solution with no additional costs and preserve QoS.

According to Mark Weiser, the creator of ubiquitous computing, "the most meaningful innovations are disappearing." Smart computing refers to a computer that enters the physical world and bridges the virtual and physical worlds. Ubiquitous computing technologies in healthcare research are oriented toward the goals of a smart, user-centered, and preventive healthcare paradigm. It is not intended to replace traditional healthcare. In comparison to traditional disease treatment, smart healthcare technologies can be employed at all phases of life to drive healthy behavior and disease prevention.

The advancement of computing power, sensors, embedded devices, smartphones, wireless communications, networking, data mining techniques, cloud computing, and social networking has prompted researchers and practitioners to develop smart computing systems that automatically respond to users in a context-aware and situation-aware manner. Smart systems must be designed to perform over a wide range of spatial and temporal scales and to include a large number of computational platforms, users, devices, and applications dealing with enormous volumes of data. Smart technology offers a wide range of applications, the most important of which is healthcare, which includes support for independent living, wellness, and illness management. Smart healthcare has the objective of assisting patients in managing their diseases as well as communicating and collaborating with healthcare specialists.

According to healthcare criteria, infrastructure should be designed in such a way that wireless technologies such as location tracking, intelligent devices, user interfaces, body sensors, and short-range wireless communications can be used effectively for health monitoring. Instant, flexible, and universal wireless connectivity can be used to boost healthcare providers' accessibility, and communication between medical devices, patients, healthcare providers, and vehicles should be reliable for effective emergency management. Current and developing wireless technologies aid in providing high-quality medical care. By improving healthcare providers' productivity, retention, and quality of life by utilizing these wireless technologies, as well as lowering the long-term cost of healthcare services.

Devices or technologies used in smart healthcare systems are very limited in energy resources. So, energy efficiency is vital for these smart healthcare services. Energy efficiency techniques suitable for these applications must be combined and designed in such a way that it meets the demands of smart healthcare systems. Since Medical Data is sensitive it should be prevented from malicious and unauthorized access or attacks. So security plays a vital role in smart healthcare services. Patient misidentification also leads to medical errors. By using smart healthcare systems these errors can be reduced.

In the future, affordability, portability, and reusability features of wireless technologies can help in reducing the overall healthcare services cost which includes health monitoring and smart healthcare service cost.

9.7 Conclusion

The main objective of the book chapter is to provide techniques for enhancing the QoS while maintaining safety in a smart healthcare system. India is moving toward being a smart nation with brilliant urban areas. Savvy social insurance is among the enormous foundations on which a shrewd nation is based. In India, quality smart healthcare services are difficult to access in smaller urban areas, towns, and towns, where most of the populace lives. Keen social insurance in India would make high-quality medicinal services accessible to every one of its subjects. Brilliant human services will likewise enhance the involvement of healthcare services for both patients and specialists.

References

1. S. Singh, S. K. Jangir, M. Kumar, M. Verma, S. Kumar, T. S. Walia, and S. M. Kamal. "Feature Importance Score-Based Functional Link Artificial Neural Networks for Breast Cancer Classification." BioMed Research International, 2022.
2. P. Bellavista, G. Cardone, A. Corradi, and L. Foschini, "Convergence of MANET and WSN in IoT urban scenarios," IEEE Sens J, 13, 10, 3558–3567, 2013.
3. A. Laya, V. I. Bratu, and J. Markendahl, "Who is investing in machine-to-machine communications?" in Proc. 24th Eur. Reg. ITS Conf., Florence, Italy, Oct. 2013, pp. 20–23.
4. H. Schaffers, N. Komninos, M. Pallot, B. Trousse, M. Nilsson, Band A. Oliveira, "Smart cities and the future internet: Towards cooperation frameworks for open innovation," The Future Internet, Lect. Notes ComputSci., vol. 6656, pp. 431–446, 2011.
5. D. Cuff, M. Hansen, and J. Kang, "Urban sensing: Out of the woods," Commun. ACM, vol. 51, no. 3, pp. 24–33, Mar. 2008.
6. M. Dohler, I. Vilajosana, X. Vilajosana, and J. Llosa, "Smart Cities: Anaction plan," in Proc. Barcelona Smart Cities Congress, Barcelona, Spain,Dec. 2011, pp. 1–6.
7. P. Chithaluru, S. Kumar, A. Singh, A. Benslimane, and S. K. Jangir. "An Energy-Efficient Routing Scheduling Based on Fuzzy Ranking Scheme for Internet of Things." IEEE Internet of Things Journal 9, no. 10 (2021): 7251–7260.
8. C. E. A. Mulligan and M. Olsson, "Architectural Implications of smart city business models: An evolutionary perspective," IEEE Commun. Mag., vol. 51, no. 6, pp. 80–85, Jun. 2013.
9. N. Walravens and P. Ballon, "Platform business models for smart cities: From control and value to governance and public value," IEEE Commun.Mag., vol. 51, no. 6, pp72–79, Jun. 2013.
10. J. P. Lynch and J. L. Kenneth, "A summary review of wireless sensors and sensor networks for structural health monitoring," Shock and VibrationDigest, vol. 38, no. 2, pp. 91–130, 2006.
11. T. Nuortio, J. Kytöjoki, H. Niska, and O. Bräysy, "Improved route planning and scheduling of waste collection and transport," Expert Syst. Appl., vol. 30, no. 2, pp. 223–232, Feb. 2006.
12. A. R. Al-Ali, I. Zualkernan, and F. Aloul, "A mobile GPRSsensors array for air pollution monitoring," IEEE Sensors J., vol. 10, no. 10, pp. 1666–1671, Oct. 2010.
13. N. Maisonneuve, M. Stevens, M. E. Niessen, P. Hanappe, and L. Steels, "Citizen noise pollution monitoring," in Proc. 10thAnnu. Int. Conf. DigitalGov. Res.: Soc. Netw.: Making Connec. Between Citizens, Data Gov., 2009, pp. 96–103.
14. X. Li, W. Shu, M. Li, H.-Y. Huang, P.-E. Luo, and M.-Y. Wu, "Performance evaluation of vehicle-based mobile sensor networks for traffic monitoring," IEEE Trans. Veh. Technol., vol. 58, no. 4, pp. 1647–1653, May 2009.
15. S. Lee, D. Yoon, and A. Ghosh, "Intelligent parking lot application using wireless sensor networks," in Proc. Int. Symp. Collab. Technol. Syst., Chicago, May 19–23, 2008, pp. 48–57.
16. W. Kastner, G. Neugschwandtner, S. Soucek, and H. M. Newmann,"Communication systems for building automation and control," in Proc.IEEE, Jun. 2005, vol. 93, no. 6, pp.1178–1203.
17. R. T Fielding, "Architectural Styles and the design of network-based software architectures," (The Representational State Transfer (REST))Ph.D. dissertation, pp 76-85, Dept. Inf. Comput. Sci. Univ. California, Irvine, 2000. [Online]. Available:http://www.ics.uci.edu/~fielding/pubs/dissertation/top.htm.
18. "Efficient XML Interchange (EXI) Format 1.0," J. Schneider, T. Kamiya, D. Peintner, and R. Kyusakov, Eds., 2nd ed. World Wide Web Consortium, Feb. 11, 2014. [Online]. Available: http://www.w3.org/TR/exi/.
19. A. P. Castellani, N. Bui, P. Casari, M. Rossi, Z. Shelby, and M. Zorzi, "Architecture and protocols for the Internet of Things: A case study," in Proc. 8th IEEE Int. Conf. Pervasive Comput. Commun. Workshops(PERCOM Workshops), 2010, pp. 678–683.
20. A. P. Castellani, M. Dissegna, N. Bui, and M. Zorzi, "WebIoT: A webapplication framework for the internet of things," in Proc. IEEE WirelessCommun. Netw. Conf. Workshops, Paris, France, 2012.

21. Z. Shelby, K. Hartke, C. Bormann, and B. Frank, the Constrained application protocol (CoAP), draft-IETF-core-cap-18 (work in progress), s.l.:IETF 2013. [Online]. Available: http://tools.ietf.org/html/draft-ietf-corecoap-18.
22. R. Sravanth, P. Chithaluru, and S. Kumar. "Eyeblink robot control using brain-computer interface for healthcare applications." International Journal of Mobile Devices, Wearable Technology, and Flexible Electronics (IJMDWTFE) 10, 2, pp 38-50, 2019.
23. Aegis Corporation. 2016. Aeris IoT services and healthcare focus on the patient. Retrieved October 12, 2016, from www.aeris.com/for-enterproses/healthcare-remote-patient-monitoring/.
24. Alera Inc. 2016. Products and Services. Retrieved October 12, 2016, from http://www.alere.com/en/home.HTML.
25. Appelboom, G., et al. 2014. Smart wearable body sensors for patient self-assessment and monitoring. Archives of Public Health 72: 28.
26. Bauer, H., M. Patel, and J. Veira. 2016. The Internet of things: Sizing up the opportunity, McKinsey. Retrieved October 12, 2016, from http://www.mckinsey.com/industries/high-tech/our-insights/the-internet-of-things-sizing-up-the-opportunity
27. Baum, S. 2015. Survey: Remote patient monitoring shifting from point solution to disease-specific, patient engagement, November 16, 2015. Retrieved October 12, 2016, from http://medcitynews.com/2015/11/remote-patient-monitoring/.
28. Bluetooth standard. 2016. Retrieved October 12, 2016, from www.bluetooth.com.
29. Cao, H., V. Leung, C. Chow, and H. Chan. 2010. Enabling technologies for wireless body area networks: A survey and outlook. IEEE Communications Magazine, 84–93.
30. Cook, D. J., J. E. Thompson, S. K. Prinsen, J. A. Dearani, and C. Deschamps. 2013. Functional recovery in the elderly after major surgery: Assessment of mobility recovery using wireless technology. Annals of Thoracic Surgery 96: 1057– 1061.
31. de Schatz, C., H. Medeiros, F. Schneider, and P. Abatti. 2012. Wireless medical sensor networks: Design requirements and enabling technologies. Telemedicine and e-Health Journal 18 (5): 394–399.
32. Di Cerbo, A., J. Morales-Medina, B. Palmieri, and T. Iannitti. 2015. A narrative review of telemedicine consultation in medical practice. Patient Preference & Adherence 9: 65–75.
33. Eurohealth. 2009. Vol. 15, No. 1, pub. London School of Economics, UK.
34. Filipe, L., F. Fdez-Riverola, N. Costa, and A. Pereira. 2015. Wireless body area network for healthcare applications: Protocol stack review. International Journal of Distributed Systems 2015 (1).
35. Plachkinova, M., S. Andres, and S. Chatterjee. 2015. A taxonomy of mHealth apps: Security and privacy concerns. Proceedings of the Hawaii International Conference on System Sciences, Hawaii, 3187–3196.
36. Qualcomm Corp. 2016. Qualcomm Life. Retrieved October 12, 2016, from https://www.qualcomm.com/news/releases/2015/01/29/Roche-and-Qualcomm-collaborate-innovate-remote-patient-monitoring.
37. Ragesh, G.K. and K. Baskaran. 2011. A survey on futuristic health care systems: WBANs. Presented at International Conference on Communication Technology and System Design, India.
38. Remote patient monitoring devices market analysis: A grand view research report. Retrieved October 12, 2016, from http://www.grandviewresearch.com/.
39. Transforming healthcare through the Internet of Things by VijayakannanSermakani, Robert Bosch Engineering and Business Ltd in 2014; pmibangalorechapter.in/pmpc/2014/tech_papers/healthcare.pdf
40. Gartner, IT Glossary, Internet of Things - http://www.gartner.com/it-glossary/internet-of-things/Gartner, Press release, 2013, online at http://www.gartner.com/newsroom/id/2636073
41. ITU Internet Reports, The Internet of Things, November 2005 http://www.itu.int/osg/spu/publications/internetofthings/InternetofThings_summary.pdf

42. ERC – European Research Cluster on the Internet of Things, "Internet of Things - Pan European Research and Innovation Vision", October 2011.
43. L. Adori, A. Iera, and G. Morabito, "The Internet of Things: A survey," in ScienceDirect: Computer Networks, vol. xx (Article in Press), pp. 1–19, May 2010.
44. H. Jun-Wei, Y. Shouyi, L. Leibo, Z. Zhen, W. Shaojun, A Crop Monitoring System Based on Wireless Sensor Network, Procedia Environmental Sciences. 11 (2011) 558–565.
45. Al-Fuqaha, M. G., et al. 2015. Internet of Things: A survey on enabling technologies, protocols, and applications. IEEE Communication Surveys and Tutorials 17 (4): 2347.
46. Bech, J. 2014. OP-TEE, Open-Source Security for the Mass-Market. Core Dump online magazine, September 3, 2014. http://www.linaro.org/blog/core-dump/op-tee-open-source-security-mass-market/.
47. Buckiewicz, B. 2016. Overview of Medical Body Area Networks, White Paper, LSR/Laird Business, Cedarburg, WI. www.lsr.com/white-papers/overview-of-medical-body-area-networks.

Chapter 10
Authentication Methods for Internet of Medical Things

10.1 Introduction

Telecare Medical Information Systems allow physicians and physicians in medical centers to remotely care for enrolled patients anywhere via the Internet. Secure and authenticated access to the medical data on the medical server is necessary in the light of patient privacy and medical data. Due to the expansion of low cost communication technology over the past few decades, telemedicine information systems have made medical services possible. With the implementation of these systems, telecare facilities that are electronically linked to computerized patient records will become more prevalent. It has greatly facilitated our lives. However, it may also contain important patient information. Authentication between the two is essential to access these services. The host server requires authentication to protect the record from unauthorized persons. You need to ensure the privacy of your patients. On the other side, since the patient must verify with the server, a hacker cannot pretend to be the server. Because of this, TMIS security is crucial. TMIS requires a more reliable and effective authentication system. Only authorized users or patients should be able to access the TMIS service, hence a secure authentication system is crucial. To achieve mutual authentication between the client and server, three authentication elements are being used. What you are aware of in the first place (usually your username and password). (b) What you possess (such as an ID card or chip card); (c) who you are (eg Biometrics).

The use of a one-way hash function to encrypt all passwords and save the digest in a validation table kept on the server is one of the most popular ways to overcome the drawbacks of validation tables. However, storing the encrypted password requires additional storage space. With this method, as the user base expands, so does the size of the validation table. The upkeep of this massive check table will put more strain on your server. Instead of using OTP, password-based smart card authentication solutions have been suggested to address these problems and

S. Gupta et al., *Blockchain for Secure Healthcare Using Internet of Medical Things (IoMT)*, https://doi.org/10.1007/978-3-031-18896-1_10

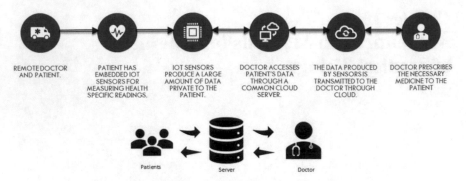

Fig. 10.1   E- Healthcare architecture

limitations. A tamper-proof integrated circuit card having memory and a processor that can conduct calculations is referred to as a smart card. The information is kept in the chip's memory and is accessible for use in a variety of processing applications. The three layers of smart card authentication techniques are listed below.

The phase of registration. When a user requests registration, the server determines the necessary parameters, stores them in the smart card's memory, and then sends the smart card to the user.

When a user attempts to log into a server, the login and authentication steps are triggered. Using the user credentials entered and the necessary settings kept in the smart card memory, the smart card generates a login request during the login process.

Authentication phase. The server verifies the login request after receiving it by verifying the requesting user's identity using its private key. The foundational structure of e-healthcare is depicted in Fig. 10.1. The smartphone receives information from the IoT sensor about the patient's physiological state. It travels through the open Internet from your smartphone to the server of your healthcare provider. Protected health information (PHI) about the patient is stored on a server, and, by the rules set by the policy server, the authentication server only permits access to the PHI following successful authentication. Areas of interest are displayed within a red block that contains users, doctors, authentication servers, and TMIS. In e-Healthcare, patients access PHI to monitor their health, doctors access prescriptions, and pharmacists access prescriptions to see what medicines are prescribed.

10.2   Authentication Schemes for Tele Medical Healthcare System

One of the most common methods to get around the limitations of validation tables is to use a one-way hash function to encrypt all passwords and save the digest in a validation table retained on the server. However, storing the encrypted password requires additional storage space. With this method, as the user base expands, so does the size of the validation table. This enormous check table will require extra maintenance, which will tax your server. Password-based smart card authentication options have been proposed as a substitute for OTP to solve these issues and restrictions. A smart card is an impenetrable integrated circuit card with memory and a CPU that can perform calculations. The data is stored on the chip and is available for use and completion. The smart card generates a login request during the login process using the user credentials entered and the appropriate parameters stored in the smart card memory [1]. The phase of authentication. The server verifies the login request after receiving it by verifying the requested user's identity using its private key. E-fundamental healthcare architecture is depicted in Fig. 10.2. The smartphone receives information from the IoT sensor about the patient's physiological state. It travels through the open Internet from your smartphone to the server of your healthcare provider. Protected health information (PHI) about the patient is stored on the storage server, and access to that PHI is only permitted upon successful authentication by the authentication server by the policies put in place by the policy server [2]. Within a block that includes users, doctors, authentication servers, and TMIS, areas of interest are displayed. Patients use PHI to track their health in e-Healthcare, doctors use prescriptions, and pharmacists use prescriptions to see what medications are recommended.

A password-based user authentication system based on hash functions, symmetric encryption, and discrete logarithm issues was proposed by Zhen et al. [3]. The phases are four. Authentication, precalculation, password-change phase, or registration. They evaluated how well their designs performed in comparison to Yang et al. [4], Xu et al. [5], and Liu et al. [6] Then he provided an effective plan that made use of eight hash functions and two exponential operations. Additionally, those plans support TMIS on low-power mobile devices. Debiao and others [7] work was

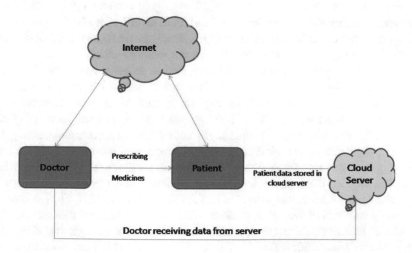

Fig. 10.2 Users and doctors use medical data stored in an IOT-cloud environment

contrasted with that of Wu et al. and Xu et al. [8, 9] and examined their strategies. The calculation time is longer since the scheme makes more use of exponential functions. Additionally, the theft of personal information hurt their goals.

To increase efficiency, Debiao et al. [7]'s methods for TMIS use only one exponential function and are compatible with low-power mobile devices. An authentication system based on forwarding Secrecy was proposed by Kahn et al. [10]. With Weietal [11], they discussed their ideas., as well as Zu et al. [12] Then he demonstrated how both strategies had issues with DoS assaults, the transfer of secrets, and password change phases. Chen [13] and others. Proposed a privacy certification program to use pairing techniques to preserve patient privacy. They also suggested using digital signatures to guarantee the privacy of medical data. Their system can withstand numerous assaults, including spoofing, replays, man-in-the-middle attacks, and security attacks on well-known keys. 18.49 s pass during the data transmission. By computing hashes and XOR functions, Mishra et al. [14] suggested an enhanced biometrics-based remote authentication approach for TMIS. With Awasthietal, they discussed their strategies [15]. And it turned out to be open to password-guessing assaults both online and offline. For use with the AVISPA tool, Amine et al. [16] suggested an effective user authentication and key exchange mechanism. They demonstrated how their system is resistant to replay and man-in-the-middle attacks using a cryptographic hash function. There are five phases to the suggested architecture. Steps of login, authentication, key sharing, medical server registration, and password update. Login and authentication have transmission costs of 768 and 1152, respectively. A plan employing the automated program ProVerif was put up by Chaudhry et al. [17] and their work was contrasted with Luetal [18]. They located Lu and co. We proposed a new and improved approach that is resistant to these attacks as this one was weak against patient anonymity compromise attacks, patient spoofing attacks, and TMIS server spoofing attacks. Communication initiatives by Chaudhry and others [17] This 140-byte technique is 140 times more effective than Lu et al. Schema (180 bytes). The elliptic Curve Cryptography-based efficiency technique was proposed by Chaudhry et al. [19]. (ECC). They contrasted their plan with the two-factor authentication system used in Islam [20]. Additionally, it was discovered to be open to user and server spoofing attacks.

Amin and others [21] a lightweight certification program based on AVISPA & Scyther was proposed. They discussed their intentions with Das and colleagues [22]. Additionally, he displayed security flaws such as patient anonymity and untraceability. Amin and co. [21]. The setup, medical server enrollment, physician server enrollment, patient enrollment, login, authentication and session key negotiation, new physician server addition, password update, and biometric update are the nine phases of this technique. Compared to Das et al. [24]'s 0.0110 ms, the whole execution cost is 0.084 ms. A three-factor authentication system based on BAN logic and AVISPA tools was provided by Chandra Kar et al. [23]. They contrasted their work with that of Wen et al. made an effort to fix the security flaws in the plan. Attacks on knowledge about temporary session keys, erroneous password updates, and inadequate authentication [23] Chandra Kar et al. This plan consists of five stages. Registration, login, authentication, password modification, and blockage of smart cards. A plan that could lower patient privacy, non-linking, message authentication, and computing expenses was put out by Chiou et al. [25]. They put a bilinear pairing-based technique into practice on their Android platform and compared it to Chenetal. unsuccessful scheme [26] as a result of the aforementioned security problems. Chiou and co. The [25] system is divided into four phases: the I Health Center Upload Phase (HUP), (ii) Patient Upload Phase (PUP), (iii) Treatment Phase (TP), and (iv) Verification Phase (CP). 2040 ms is the total price for all phases. Chaudhry and others [27] We have suggested a secure and compact method utilizing ProVerif (a verification tool). Three pieces: I Description (ii) Process (iii) most crucial. Among other things, they have amines [28]. The plan proved to be impervious to attacks using stolen validators and smart cards. Their strategy consists of five steps. Logging in, authenticating, changing passwords, and a password recovery step. With Amin et al., execution time and communication costs are compared. 1.63 ms and 1664 bits. Either 2048 bits or 24.54 ms. The technique is resistant to attacks like efficient password changing, mutual authentication, and session key negotiation. A dynamic identity-based authentication technique based on BAN logic was presented by Chaturvedi Di et al. [29]. Their system thwarts attempts to guess offline passwords. In the step where the password was changed, the scheme discovered an invalid input. Registration, login, authentication, and password change are the four steps in their plan. In comparison to Chen et al., the communication overhead is 1280 bits [30]. 960-bit scheme A plan that offers forward security and resistance to Key Compromise Impersonation (KCI) assaults were put forth by Chen et al. [31]. With Chiou et al., they compared their plans [32]. It was also found to be vulnerable to KCI and forward security attacks. They used a bilinear pairing operation and a random oracle model to calculate the computational cost. In contrast to Chiouetal's 2.0955 s, this took 2.3479 s.

To Hsu et al. [34], Amin et al. [33] offered a mutual authentication system utilizing bilinear pairing and AVISPA, however, it was unsuccessful due to the aforementioned security flaw during simulation and security validation. Their research was contrasted with that of Hsu et al. [34], who employed bilinear pairing and ECC. Their plan was broken down into six stages: user registration, login, authentication & session key agreement, password changing, and password recovery. Their plan takes 45.97 ms to execute as opposed to the 22.05 ms plan of Hsu et al. They asserted that the Hsu et al. technique failed to withstand an offline password guessing attack. Although their plan defeated all of these attacks, it had drawbacks including a slow response time and hefty processing costs.

A lightweight authentication method that protects patients' anonymity and thwarts attacks on stolen mobile devices was created by Mohit et al. [35]. They demonstrated that their system does not support mobile device theft assaults and patient confidentiality by contrasting it with Chiou et al. [36]'s work. The healthcare center upload phase, patient data upload phase, treatment phase, and check-up phase are the four phases of the scheme, according to Mohit et al. [35]. When compared to the Mohit et al. [35] system, the execution time of the Chiou et al. (2.086 ms). When compared to Mohit et al. scheme, Chiou et al. approach had a higher communication cost (6528 bits) (5312 bits).

To offer excellent performance and efficiency, Irshad et al. [37] suggested a multi-server authentication technique based on BAN logic. They proposed three phases: registration, login and authentication, and password modification. They used ECC. The suggested technique takes 26.8 ms to execute. They contrasted their plan with that of Amin et al. [38], which was susceptible to attacks such as password guessing and impersonating.

In their review paper, Aslam et al. [39] examined earlier studies on 1-factor, 2-factor, and 3-factor authentication methods. For one factor, the performance metric security index was utilized, while for two and three factors, the performance metric security index was combined with user computation cost, server computation cost, user & server efficiency, and security index. The hybrid approach that was suggested provided 3-factor authentication for doctors and 2-factor authentication for patients.

Reduced redundancy in the design of the authentication process was offered by Li Chun et al. [40] to secure the transfer of sensor data. The data in an IoT-based medical care system was encrypted by Li Chun et al. [40] using the random oracle approach. They proposed five phases, setup, registration, login, verification & access control, and encryption, and they compared their article with Liu Chung et al. [41]'s work. Their plan's execution takes 3:51 ms as opposed to Liu Chung's plan's 13.81 ms. Their plan was resistant to several assaults, including password revelation, replay password guessing, data forgery, sensed data leak, and smart card theft.

The BAN logic model was used by Mishra et al. [42] to provide a strong authentication technique in WSN. Their plan consists of six steps, including the registration of sensor nodes and gateway nodes, users, logins, authentication, password changes, and the addition of sensor nodes. Their plan might withstand user anonymity, off-line passwords, insider attacks by privileged individuals, smartcard theft, user impersonation, and replay attacks. It employs symmetric key encryption, a hash function, and public-key cryptographic operations. A total of 16,384 bits are used in communication.

An enhanced two-factor authentication system based on the Oracle model and BAN logic was presented by Xiong et al. [43]. Their plan can withstand a variety of harmful assaults, including Replay, user anonymity, man-in-the-middle, offline dictionaries, and privileged insider attacks. They contend that their plan is more dependable and effective.

Rotating group signatures were utilized by Mehmood et al. [44] and were based on Elliptic Curve Cryptography (ECC). For added protection, they also made use of "The Onion Router (TOR)". They talked about the drawbacks of earlier research, such as PKC (Public Key Cryptosystem), which was impractical for mobile networks. Schemes based on pseudonyms were unsuccessful due to high computational expense. Without disclosing the patient's identity, their plan protected their privacy.

To enable patients to remotely access medical services in confidence, Zhang et al. [45] developed a telemedical information model based on cloud authentication. It consists of four phases: the uploading phase for the healthcare center, the patient upload phase, the treatment phase, and the checking report phase. Their system offers both message authentication and data secrecy. Additionally, their plan offers greater computation cost efficiency.

A dependable energy-efficient method was put out by Liu et al. [46] employing an elliptic curve discrete logarithmic issue. They contrasted their study with Cheng et al. [47], which had security problems with patient anonymity and communication confidentiality. The five phases of the approach they proposed—patient registration, healthcare center upload, patient upload, therapy, and checking up—performed better and required less calculation.

To address problems common to wireless sensor networks, Quanet et al. [48] presented an identity-based cryptographic authentication approach. Due to its deployment in an open environment, WSN's sensor nodes are vulnerable to numerous attacks, which causes issues with user authentication. Five phases—registration, user registration, login and authentication, authentication, and password update—were proposed by the authors as a mechanism for data collection through sensor networks.

Two tools, AVISPA and Scyther, were proposed as part of an authentication strategy by Amin et al. [49]. They demonstrated that their approach could withstand patient confidentiality and intractability by comparing it to Das et al. [50]'s scheme. In comparison to the method proposed by Das et al., Amin et al. [49]'s scheme was more effective and trustworthy because it was based on cryptography and hash functions.

An authentication method based on the El-Gamal cryptosystem, which can withstand 14 attacks, was proposed by Salem et al. Salem et al. demonstrated the effectiveness of their plan by simulating it using the AVISPA program [51]. To read, write, and acquire data from a tag, they employed robust and reusable RFID technology. A tag for the uniqueness feature and a card reader for memory space, encryption, and decryption modules were their two main suggestions.

For IoT-based WBANs, Vijayakumar et al. [52]'s suggested authentication technique maintains location privacy. The authors offered a framework for anonymously authenticating both the doctor and the patient. In WBAN, [54] et al. have specified their effort (Wireless Body Area Networks). Their plan protects both patients' and physicians' privacy and integrity. Additionally, they suggested a six-phase WBAN strategy to ban disruptive users.

The three primary types of IoMT's current authentication protocols can be separated based on the cryptosystem. There are symmetric cryptosystem-based, asymmetric cryptosystem-based, and hybrid protocols, as depicted in Fig. 10.3. A safe cryptographic hash function is used by the majority of authentication schemes.

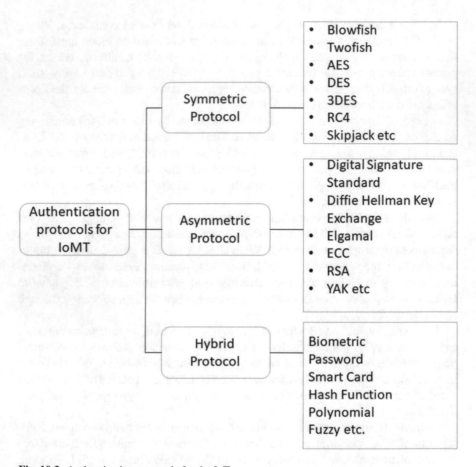

Fig. 10.3 Authentication protocols for the IoT

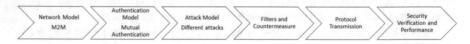

Fig. 10.4 Process of authentication protocol

10.3   Processes of an Authentication Protocol

A method of authentication developed especially for use in electronic medical records. The IoT authentication protocol implementation is built on the strategy depicted in Fig. 10.4, which is:

1. An explanation of a network model (e.g. M2M, IoV, IoE, IoS).
2. Definition of the authentication model (mutual authentication, complete transfer secrecy, anonymity, untraceable, etc.).

3. Third specification of an assault model (e.g. replay attack, stolen smart card attack, privileged insider attack, offline password guessing attack, spoofing attack, sensor node capture attack).
4. Defenses are chosen (e.g. encryption methods, Bloom filters, biometrics, smart cards, access polynomials, and Chebyshev chaos maps).
5. Suggestions for the main aspects of the protocol (e.g. initialization, registration process).
6. Formal security evaluation employing security analysis (e.g., ProVerif, BAN-logic, AVISPA) (e.g. ProVerif, BAN-logic, AVISPA).
7. Performance assessment (e.g. storage cost, computational complexity, communication overhead, reduced error rate, etc.).

10.4   Conclusion

This chapter covered the various WMSN authentication procedures. With the assistance of the Internet of Things and cloud computing, this system enables patients to access health monitoring and services over the Internet. Saving time and money on travel and patient care is a goal of TMHS. A detailed and organized overview of IoT authentication techniques is provided in this white paper. Depending on the target environment, these logs can be categorized. Future directions for research are established in light of this analysis. As long as they can collaborate with other systems to recognize and stop IoT threats, IoT authentication protocols can protect both authentication and privacy, making them more effective in terms of computing complexity and communication overhead.

References

1. Kumari, S., & Khan, M. K. More secure smart card-based remote user password authentication scheme with user anonymity. Secure. Communications and Network, 7, 2039–2053, 2013. https://doi.org/10.1002/sec.916
2. Kumari, S., Khan, M. K., & Kumar, R. Cryptanalysis and improvement of a privacy-enhanced scheme for telecare medical information systems. Journal of Medical Systems, 37(4), 9952, 2013. https://doi.org/10.1007/s10916-013-9952-5
3. Wu ZY, Lee YC, Lai F, Lee HC, Chung Y. A secure authentication scheme for telecare medicine information systems. J Med Syst. 2012 Jun;36(3):1529-35. doi: https://doi.org/10.1007/s10916-010-9614-9. Epub 2010 Oct 27.
4. Yang, C. C., Wang, R. C., and Liu, W. T., Secure authentication scheme for session initiation protocol. Comput. Secure. 24:381–386, 2005.
5. Xu, J., Zhu, W. T., and Feng, D. G., An improved smart card-based password authentication scheme with provable security. Comput. Stand. Interfaces 31(4):723–728, 2009.
6. Liu, J. Y., Zhou, A. M., and Gao, M. X., A new mutual authentication scheme based on nonce and smart cards. Comput. Commun. 31(10):2205–2209, 2008.

7. Debiao, H., Jianhua, C., & Rui, Z. (2011). A More Secure Authentication Scheme for Telecare Medicine Information Systems. Journal of Medical Systems, 36(3), 1989–1995. doi:https://doi.org/10.1007/s10916-011-9658-5

8. Xu, J., Zhu, W. T., and Feng, D. G., An improved smart card-based password authentication scheme with provable security. Comput. Stand. Interfaces 31(4):723–728, 2009.

9. Wu, Z.-Y., Lee, Y.-C., Lai, F., Lee H.-C., and Chung, Y., A Secure Authentication Scheme for Telecare Medicine Information Systems. J. Med. Syst. doi:https://doi.org/10.1007/s10916-010-9614-9.

10. Khan, M. K., & Kumari, S. (2013). An Authentication Scheme for Secure Access to Healthcare Services. Journal of Medical Systems, 37(4). doi:https://doi.org/10.1007/s10916-013-9954-3

11. Wei, J., Hu, X., and Liu, W., An improved authentication scheme for telecare medicine information systems. J. Med. Syst. 36(6):3597–3604, 2012. doi:https://doi.org/10.1007/s10916-012-9835-1.

12. Zhu, Z., An efficient authentication scheme for telecare medicine information systems. J. Med. Syst. 36(6):3833–3838, 2012. doi:https://doi.org/10.1007/s10916-012-9856-9.

13. Chen, C.-L., Yang, T.-T., Chiang, M.-L., & Shih, T.-F. (2014). A Privacy Authentication Scheme Based on Cloud for Medical Environment. Journal of Medical Systems, 38(11). doi:https://doi.org/10.1007/s10916-014-0143-9

14. Mishra, D., Mukhopadhyay, S., Kumari, S., Khan, M. K., & Chaturvedi, A. (2014). Security Enhancement of a Biometric based Authentication Scheme for Telecare Medicine Information Systems with Nonce. Journal of Medical Systems, 38(5). doi:https://doi.org/10.1007/s10916-014-0041-1

15. Awasthi, A. K., and Srivastava, K., A biometric authentication scheme for telecare medicine information systems with nonce. J. Med. Syst. 37(5):1–4, 2013.

16. Amin, R., & Biswas, G. P. (2015). A Novel User Authentication and Key Agreement Protocol for Accessing Multi-Medical Server Usable in TMIS. Journal of Medical Systems, 39(3). doi:https://doi.org/10.1007/s10916-015-0217-3

17. Chaudhry, S. A., Mahmood, K., Naqvi, H., & Khan, M. K. (2015). An Improved and Secure Biometric Authentication Scheme for Telecare Medicine Information Systems Based on Elliptic Curve Cryptography. Journal of Medical Systems, 39(11). doi:https://doi.org/10.1007/s10916-015-0335-y

18. Lu, Y., Li, L., Peng, H., and Yang, Y., An enhanced biometric based authentication scheme for telecare medicine information systems using elliptic curve cryptosystem. J. Med. Syst. 39(3):1–8, 2015.

19. Chaudhry, S. A., Naqvi, H., Shon, T., Sher, M., &Farash, M. S. (2015). Cryptanalysis and Improvement of an Improved Two Factor Authentication Protocol for Telecare Medical Information Systems. Journal of Medical Systems, 39(6). doi:https://doi.org/10.1007/s10916-015-0244-0

20. Islam, S., and Khan, M., Cryptanalysis and improvement of authentication and key agreement protocols for telecare medicine information systems. J. Med. Syst. 38(10):135, 2014. doi:https://doi.org/10.1007/s10916-014-0135-9.

21. Amin, R., Islam, S. H., Gope, P., Choo, K.-K. R., & Tapas, N. (2018). Anonymity preserving and Lightweight Multi-Medical Server Authentication Protocol for Telecare Medical Information System. IEEE Journal of Biomedical and Health Informatics, 1–1. doi:https://doi.org/10.1109/jbhi.2018.2870319

22. Das, A. K., Odelu, V., & Goswami, A. (2015). "A secure and robust user authenticated key agreement scheme for hierarchical multi-medical server environment in TMIS", Journal of medical systems, 39(9), 92

23. Chandrakar, P., & Om, H. (2016). Cryptanalysis and Extended Three-Factor Remote User Authentication Scheme in Multi-Server Environment. Arabian Journal for Science and Engineering, 42(2), 765–786. doi:https://doi.org/10.1007/s13369-016-2341-x

24. Wen, F.; Susilo, W.; Yang, G.: Analysis and improvement on a biometric-based remote user authentication scheme using smart cards. Wirel. Personal Commun. 80(4), 1747–1760 (2015)

25. Chiou, S.-Y., Ying, Z., & Liu, J. (2016). Improvement of a Privacy Authentication Scheme Based on Cloud for Medical Environment. Journal of Medical Systems, 40(4). doi:https://doi.org/10.1007/s10916-016-0453-1

26. Chen, C. L., Yang, T. T., Chiang, M. L., and Shih, T. F., A Privacy Authentication Scheme Based on Cloud for Medical Environment. J. Med. Syst. 38:143, 2014. doi:https://doi.org/10.1007/s10916-014-0143-9.

27. Chaudhry, S. A., Khan, M. T., Khan, M. K., & Shon, T. (2016). A Multiserver Biometric Authentication Scheme for TMIS using Elliptic Curve Cryptography. Journal of Medical Systems, 40(11). doi:https://doi.org/10.1007/s10916-016-0592-4

28. Amin, R., Islam, S. H., Biswas, G., Khan, M. K., and Kumar, N., An efficient and practical smart card based anonymity preserving user authentication scheme for tmis using elliptic curve cryptography. J Med Syst 39(11):1–18, 2015

29. Chaturvedi, A., Mishra, D., & Mukhopadhyay, S. (2017). An enhanced dynamic ID-based authentication scheme for telecare medical information systems. Journal of King Saud University - Computer and Information Sciences, 29(1), 54–62. doi: https://doi.org/10.1016/j.jksuci.2014.12.007

30. Chen, H.-M., Lo, J.-W., Yeh, C.-K., 2012. An efficient and secure dynamic id-based authentication scheme for telecare medical information systems. J. Med. Syst. 36 (6), 3907–3915.

31. Cheng, Q., Zhang, X., & Ma, J. (2017). ICASME: An Improved Cloud-Based Authentication Scheme for Medical Environment. Journal of Medical Systems, 41(3). doi:https://doi.org/10.1007/s10916-017-0693-8

32. Chiou, S. Y., Ying, Z., and Liu, J., Improvement of a Privacy Authentication Scheme Based on Cloud for Medical Environment. J. Med. Syst. 40(4):1–15, 2016

33. Amin, R., Islam, S. H., Vijayakumar, P., Khan, M. K., & Chang, V. (2017). A robust and efficient bilinear pairing based mutual authentication and session key verification over insecure communication. Multimedia Tools and Applications, 77(9), 11041–11066. doi:https://doi.org/10.1007/s11042-017-4996-z

34. Hsu CL, Chuang YH, Kuo CL (2015) A novel remote user authentication scheme from bilinear pairings via internet. WirelPersCommun 83(1):163–174

35. Mohit, P., Amin, R., Karati, A., Biswas, G. P., & Khan, M. K. (2017). A Standard Mutual Authentication Protocol for Cloud Computing Based Health Care System. Journal of Medical Systems, 41(4). doi:https://doi.org/10.1007/s10916-017-0699-2

36. Chiou, S. Y., Ying, Z., and Liu, J., Improvement of a privacy authentication scheme based on cloud for medical environment. J. Med. Syst. 40(4):1–15, 2016

37. Irshad, A., Sher, M., Nawaz, O., Chaudhry, S. A., Khan, I., & Kumari, S. (2016). A secure and provable multi-server authenticated key agreement for TMIS based on Amin et al..scheme. Multimedia Tools and Applications, 76(15), 16463–16489. doi:https://doi.org/10.1007/s11042-016-3921-1

38. Amin R, Islam SH, Biswas GP, Khan MK, Kumar N (2015) An efficient and practical smart card based anonymity preserving user authentication scheme for TMIS using elliptic curve cryptography. J Med Syst 39(11):1–18

39. Aslam, M. U., Derhab, A., Saleem, K., Abbas, H., Orgun, M., Iqbal, W., & Aslam, B. (2016). A Survey of Authentication Schemes in Telecare Medicine Information Systems. Journal of Medical Systems, 41(1). doi:https://doi.org/10.1007/s10916-016-0658-3

40. Li, C.-T., Wu, T.-Y., Chen, C.-L., Lee, C.-C., & Chen, C.-M. (2017). An Efficient User Authentication and User Anonymity Scheme with Provably Security for IoT-Based Medical Care System. Sensors, 17(7), 1482. doi:https://doi.org/10.3390/s17071482

41. Liu, C.H.; Chung, Y.F. Secure user authentication scheme for wireless healthcare sensor networks. Comput. Electr. Eng. 2016, 59, 250–261, doi: https://doi.org/10.1016/j.compeleceng.2016.01.002.

42. Mishra, D., Vijayakumar, P., Sureshkumar, V., Amin, R., Islam, S. H., &Gope, P. (2017). Efficient authentication protocol for secure multimedia communications in IoT-enabled wireless sensor networks. Multimedia Tools and Applications, 77(14), 18295–18325. doi:https://doi.org/10.1007/s11042-017-5376-4

43. Xiong, H., Tao, J., & Yuan, C. (2017). Enabling Telecare Medical Information Systems with Strong Authentication and Anonymity. IEEE Access, 1–1. doi:https://doi.org/10.1109/access.2017.2678104

44. Mehmood, A., Natgunanathan, I., Xiang, Y., Poston, H., & Zhang, Y. (2018). Anonymous Authentication Scheme for Smart Cloud Based Healthcare Applications. IEEE Access, 6, 33552–33567. doi:https://doi.org/10.1109/access.2018.2841972

45. Wenmin Li,1 ShuoZhang, 1 Qi Su,2 Qiaoyan Wen,1 and Yang Chen1, "An Anonymous Authentication Protocol Based on Cloud for Telemedical Systems", Hindawi, Wireless Communications and Mobile Computing Volume 2018, Article ID 8131367, 12 pages https://doi.org/10.1155/2018/8131367

46. Liu, X., & Ma, W. (2018). ETAP: Energy-Efficient and Traceable Authentication Protocol in Mobile Medical Cloud Architecture. IEEE Access, 6, 33513–33528. doi:https://doi.org/10.1109/access.2018.2841004

47. Q Cheng Q, X Zhang, J Ma. ICASME: An improved cloud based authentication scheme for medical environment [J]. Journal of medical systems, vol. 41, no. 3, pp: 23-44, 2017.

48. Quan, Z., Chunming, T., Xianghan, Z., &Chunming, R. (2015). A secure user authentication protocol for sensor network in data capturing. Journal of Cloud Computing, 4(1). doi:https://doi.org/10.1186/s13677-015-0030-z

49. Amin, R., Islam, S. H., Gope, P., Choo, K.-K. R., & Tapas, N. (2018). Anonymity preserving and Lightweight Multi-Medical Server Authentication Protocol for Telecare Medical Information System. IEEE Journal of Biomedical and Health Informatics, 1–1. doi:https://doi.org/10.1109/jbhi.2018.2870319

50. Das, A. K., Odelu, V., & Goswami, A. (2015). "A secure and robust user authenticated key agreement scheme for hierarchical multi-medical server environment in TMIS", Journal of medical systems, 39(9), 92

51. Fatty M. Salem, Ruhul Amin, A privacy-preserving RFID authentication protocol based on El-Gamal cryptosystem for secure TMIS, InformationSciences, Volume 527,2020, Pages 382–393,ISSN 0020-0255,https://doi.org/10.1016/j.ins.2019.07.029.

52. P. Vijayakumar, M. S. Obaidat, M. Azees, S. H. Islam and N. Kumar, "Efficient and Secure Anonymous Authentication With Location Privacy for IoT-Based WBANs," in IEEE Transactions on Industrial Informatics, vol. 16, no. 4, pp. 2603–2611, April 2020, doi: https://doi.org/10.1109/TII.2019.2925071.

Chapter 11
Blockchain-Based EHR Storage and Access Control System

11.1 Introduction

The blockchain technology has been into existence since 1991. A group of researchers had an aim for themselves, as they tried to solve the problem of tampering essential digital documents particularly, by the means of timestamping. However, when it comes to a major breakthrough, it was done by Satoshi Nakamoto in the year 2009 [1]. He used this technology for the purpose of creating digital cryptocurrency bitcoin. Since then, fields in which it has been applied has increased manifold. However, before diving into the endless applications that it offers us, it is essential that we understand all the basics and features of this technology. Blockchain is said to be have a peer-to-peer network which is decentralized and has ledger that is distributed to everyone that is a part of that network. Also, blockchain networks are open to anyone to become a part of and start availing the various benefits. Every block in the blockchain stores essential information that corresponds to the transactions that take place, pertaining to various use cases. Now that we know that blockchain stores data in blocks, we will understand a block and its contents in detail. So, every block that is a part of the blockchain contains some general basic information, which includes data, a unique hash value for the current block, a unique hash value of the previous block. Every block may contain same number of transactions, or different number of transactions. The first block that is a part of the blockchain is termed as the Genesis Block. It completely depends on the organization who is managing the blockchain network. Also, the hash of every block has to be unique, secure and irreversible. In case there is a hash function that can be easily identified, reversed, or has multiple collisions (same hash value for two different inputs), it will create a huge problem on the security aspect of the blockchain network. Thus, SHA-256 algorithm [2, 4] is used generally.

S. Gupta et al., *Blockchain for Secure Healthcare Using Internet of Medical Things (IoMT)*, https://doi.org/10.1007/978-3-031-18896-1_11

- The type of data stored, for example, documents or data such as medical data, varies according to the use case, and thus is based on the type of blockchain that is created. For example, every block in the bitcoin blockchain will store some basic general information, such as the data regarding the sender, receiver, and transaction amount, however, it may vary according to every application and use case for which it is put to use.
- The hash uniquely identifies every block in the blockchain. The calculation of hash for each and every block will be done by taking into consideration the contents that are stored in the block. Through this we can understanding that changing the contents of the block will lead to change in the hash of the block. Now since every block will contain a hash value of the block that is before it (except for genesis block) [3], so a change in the value of hash will occur because of a change in block data, thus affecting the entire ledger. This entire process will occur because of the change in value of the hash of previous block will cause a change in the hash value for all the blocks that are further aligned in the blockchain. This concept is thus used in identifying the tampered data and blocks in the blockchain.

11.1.1   Security

Now we have understood the basic concepts of a blockchain and all of its components. Let's apprehend what makes blockchain so secure. Imagine if someone changes the data inside a block. This action will result in a change of the hash value of that block, along with all the subsequent blocks as discussed in the above sections. But what if the person tries to solve this problem by recalculating the hash for all the block that were affected, thus trying to validate the tampered blockchain? This could result in questioning of the security of our data. So to prevent something like this from happening, it is seen that it takes about 10 min to make a new block from scratch [5]. Not only does it require a significant amount of time, but it also requires a high amount of computation power. A normal daily use laptops or pcs would not be compatible enough to perform computations that require such high power and system configurations. Thus, only some specific people, known as Miners, who are a part of the system are allowed to validate a set of transactions that will be included in the block, and then make the block a part of the entire blockchain. So, completing the entire process would take almost forever for all the blocks in the chain to get validated. Apart from this, a new block is added to the chain only when approved by more than 50% of the peers. Since it is impossible to change the blocks for more than 50% of the people, there is zero probability of any swindle with transactions. Thus, we can safely infer the fact that the blockchain technology supports a network which is based on peer-to-peer connection and it helps us in eliminating the need for any intermediates who otherwise might have been involved in the various transactions processes (Fig. 11.1).

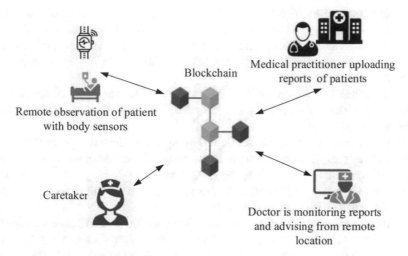

Fig. 11.1 Blockchain in smart healthcare

Apart from the above-mentioned point, an important concept of blockchain is digital signature, which is implemented using the keys pairs. Whenever a user becomes a part of the system, he/she is provided with a key pair, that includes a public key and a private key. There are various possible algorithms for creating a key pair, such as RSA (Rivest-Shamir-Adleman encryption algorithm) [6, 9], etc. The private key will be visible only to the user to which it belongs, and no one else. This private key is used to perform all the transactions. Every transaction is said to be a combination of the transaction message, that may include the name of the sender, receiver, amount to be donated and some information which would be specific to the use case, along with the private key of the sender. Thus, no transaction is possible in the name of the user, without him knowing it, because only he is aware of his private key. This combination of transaction message and private key of the user is also known as Digital Signature. Through this point, we can again emphasize on the fact that blockchain is a secure system which can be trusted for all the transactions that take place through it.

11.1.2   Features

With the advancements in the technology, people have started using it at a larger scale in industries that range in almost all fields. A few features or benefits of adopting this technology include:

- Blockchain offers a high level of transparency, as every user who is a part of the system owns a copy of all the transactions that have taken place since the start, till the current date. Thus, there is a very high level of transparency in transactions and communications [7]. This helps in developing a greater trust in the users of this technology.
- It eliminates the requirement of intermediates like banks or companies that ensure that the trades take place as intended. Thus, it fulfils the requirements of being decentralized.
- In the conventional methods, the details of all transactions are sorted in the database of any particular organization. But through this technology, every participant in the blockchain has a copy of the entire transaction history, also known as the **ledger**. It is based on the above mentioned facts that the blockchain technology is said to have a distributed ledger [8].
- As mentioned earlier, it offers a high level of security for all the transactions that take place. All transactions are said to be immutable, that is, they cannot be altered. People with any level of authority, be it administrators also do not have the rights to alter or delete any transactions.

11.2   Types of Blockchain Networks

Blockchain is implemented in a peer-to-peer network. However, there are four major ways in which the network can be created. They include:

11.2.1   Public Blockchain Network

This is a type of network which is open to all. Anyone who wishes to become a part of the network is free to do so. Example of such a blockchain network is Bitcoin. With such an open level of participation, a high overhead cost is incurred. This is because, the computation power that is required is quite high, with a little less level of security [10].

11.2.2   Private Blockchain Network

This network is similar to the public blockchain network, however, there is a single organization that keeps a check on the entire network, by restricting the people who are allowed to participate and maintaining the ledger which includes the details of all the transactions. Thus, it ensures a higher level of security and trust amongst people.

11.2.3 Permissioned Blockchain Network

This is a type of network which is open to all, however, anyone who wishes to be a part of it would require a to join the particular blockchain network, failing which, entry would be simply denied. This helps in keeping a check on the people who are a part of the network [11]. Thus, this can be used by private blockchain networks as well.

11.2.4 Consortium Blockchain Networks

Whenever there are multiple organizations that are a part of the network, and they decide to share the various responsibilities of maintaining the blockchain and the network, it is these organizations that have the rights to decide the people who will be able to perform the transactions as well as have access to the essential data that needs to be shared [12].

11.3 Applications of Blockchain

The above discussion brings us to the end of basics and benefits of using the block-chain technology. With such benefits and features, it is no wonder that there are various organizations across various fields that have already adopted the blockchain technology. The details and scope will be discussed in the further sections.

11.3.1 Smart Contracts

As the name suggests, are the contracts that involve blockchain into them, thus adding more benefits and security features. Smart contracts are similar to the normal contracts, however, they eliminate the need of any third party organizations or middlemen which is not only responsible for increasing the accountability and trust in a directly proportional fashion, but it also helps in reducing the cost by eliminating middlemen and other organizations. A list of use cases that are associated with smart contracts include offering automatic payments by banks, processing of claims by various insurance companies, and tracking payments during delivery by postal companies. Some of the use cases to understand in detail includes storing as well as transferring of sensitive medical data of various patients. This use case can be further extended to displaying and storing of the personalized healthcare report of every user or patient and sharing it with doctors and other professionals for further use as well. Apart from this use case, a company name Mediachain focusses on providing musicians and various other artists with the money and financial benefits that they should get in reality, that is, whatever they truly deserve. Through the transparent contracts, they can get their full payment instantaneously, and they may also get greater royalties. This can also be extended to tracking certain music rights for various artists. Another use case which is widely used is using the blockchain network to issue titles against the land that they buy. By introducing blockchain into the registry system, a very secure storage of information is promised. One of the company that is using this technique already is Propy [13], which is located in California.

11.3.2   Involving Blockchain into Internet of Things (IOT)

We are well aware of IOT being the new hype amongst people when it comes to upcoming technologies that will have a major impact. IOT has various applications, which are increasing till date. Many people have started adopting this technology. Thus, when we talk about a technology at such a large scale, we should also consider the security aspects. IOT [14, 15] is accustomed to face various cyber security threats. By involving Blockchain into IOT, we can securely store, monitor and alter the huge amounts of data that is generated by every device that is in use. For example, using a centralized system or server that stores essential data, such as passwords make it threat prone. Thus, by involving blockchain in this IOT based system, there will be no such central server and the end product will include biometric solutions instead of passwords. This, it will prevent the IOT devices in use to be hacked in any possible way.

11.3.3   Preventing Identity Theft

The number of cases that report identity theft is increasing day by day. There are various ways in which this can happen, which includes, stealing of personal data such as birth certificates, voter ID cards etc., through various websites, obtaining forged documents that may include aadhar or card pan which are used to pay taxes, credit card details or even account details of various OTT platforms [16], through dark web or any other available method. Also, people knowingly provide or upload fake documents for validation at times, and there are chances that they might not get caught. Thus, this problem can be solved if we start storing all the legitimate documents that are unique for a person, into the blockchain network. In case a person tries to upload fake documents, the hash of the current document will not match with the hash to the legit document that is uploaded on the network. Thus, this will not only help us in identifying any case where people get away by uploading fake documents, it also eliminates the possibility of any forgery. This initiative has also been already implemented by the government of Illinois.

11.4   Application of Blockchain in Smart Healthcare

The healthcare industry is responsible for the wellbeing of all the people in our nation. It is need of the hour that we understand it and move away from the traditional ways of working, and include other technologies as well, so that the trust of people remains intact by avoiding anything that might be incorrect or prone to errors or might get tampered.

By the involvement of various technologies such as blockchain, we can transform our healthcare system into a smart healthcare system. The various ways in which we can this can be done includes:

11.4.1   Keeping Transparency in Delivering Healthcare Goods

People buying medical goods have the right to know the information about their goods being manufactured, and how are they delivered at every stage. However, there is no proper way in which they can get this information. This problem can be solved by the introduction of blockchain by creating a system which will track our medical product at every stage, that it goes through. This information can be shared with the users as per their request. This will not only help in providing a transparent tracking system for users, but also help in reducing thousands of deaths that occur annually due to consumption of medicines that are fit for consumption due to various reasons. Also, in case any issue is spotted during the chain, it will also be rectified there and then itself, thus avoiding any manual errors and delay [16].

11.4.2   Storing of Medical Data of Patients

It is a well-known fact that a huge amount of data is generated in the medical industry. However, keeping a proper record of every patient and the medical history that they hold has been a major challenge since long. In fact, lack of history of the patient might even lead to death in the worst case scenario, and has been the case for many individuals. By looking closely, we can understand that this is a problem that can be resolved once we include the blockchain technology. The blockchain network can be added to the existing medical records of the patients, thus merging them to form a single platform to retrieve data. Patients will have full knowledge about their information being updated or shared with any doctor, professional or organization for that matter. Any document, such as a prescription or report will be added to the network by the creation of a unique hash for it, which will be updated to the user, and consent will be received.

11.4.3 Remote Health Monitoring Using IOT and Blockchain

With the advent of pandemic, which was so uncertain for anyone, the daily treatment of many people have suffered. Patients who needed daily therapies were unable to receive them on time. So to tackle such a situation, remote healthcare would be the best possible situation. There are various IOT devices available in the market that can be used to track the heart rate, blood pressure, sugar etc. This data has to be sent to doctors and professionals but ensure security as well. The security of this data and confidentiality can be ensured by the utilization of blockchain for storing and transferring of this data. Through transfer of this data at regular intervals, we can monitor it, which can be used by doctors to predict any unusual reaction, thus predicting the problem well in advance.

When we talk about the future scope of this technology, there is one essential thing to understand first. Blockchain is more like a science that needs a lot of research. It might take a few years to for this technology to reach its potential level. Also, it will emerge along with other technologies like the Internet of things or Artificial Intelligence and Machine learning, which will allow us to simplify various redundant or demanding tasks. The day is not very far away when we might not be able to imagine living our lives without the use of this technology! Who knows? The future remains uncertain.

11.5 Electronic Health Record (EHR) and Its Storage

11.5.1 Medical Big Data Mining and Processing in e-Healthcare

Medical services gained its present impact with respect to huge information innovation because of the way that the information sources associated with medical services are notable for their volume, heterogeneous intricacy, and high dynamism. With regards to huge information, the achievement of medical services applications relies exclusively upon the fundamental design and usage of proper instruments, as proven in spearheading research endeavours. Large information innovation has numerous areas of utilization in medical care, for example, prescient displaying and clinical choice help, sickness or wellbeing reconnaissance, general wellbeing, and exploration. Huge information examination in medication and medical services covers incorporation and investigation of a lot of complicated heterogeneous biomedical information and electronic wellbeing records information. Since the volume of information is immense, it should be utilized as a benefit to give the perfect mediation at the ideal time and build up customized care for the patients. Subsequently this helps all parts of the medical care framework. This section means to give a superior medical care structure tackling the advantages of enormous information investigation. The gigantic clinical information is handled viably by utilizing different logical instruments, in this way showing up at more profound experiences into the information. The current frameworks utilize calculations like fake neural organizations, strategic relapse, and fluffy based calculations [16]. A few strategies involved multitude advancement for order. The bunching involved utilization of self-coordinating guides and k-implies. This section proposes another structure for medical services involving support vector machines and examines the exhibition for large information as far as exactness, awareness, mistake rate, and region under the ROC bend. The proposed framework is.

contrasted and the ordinary framework as far as RMSE and MAPE esteem and the outcomes demonstrate promising for the recently proposed framework.

11.5.2   Smart Healthcare Systems Using Big Data

Electronic health records (EHR) are one more boundless use of huge information instruments and Techniques in the wellbeing area. Customized records incorporate traits like individual data, clinical history, obsessive tests, sensitivities, touchy sickness, and so on Clinical records are moved by means of a solid and safe medium and each clinical record is editable by a specialist. All the alters in the first record are saved with no security risk while information consistency and uprightness are likewise made do with large information examination. EHRs can likewise be utilized to send alerts and suggestions to a patient.

11.6   Significance of Blockchain in Security of Electronic Health Record (EHR)

Blockchain is a concept that facilitates the execution of transactions between two or more parties in a trustworthy manner, without the requirement for a validating or trust authority in the middle. Transacting or executing instructions no longer necessitates using a previously required tier. Every node on the network has a copy of the data so that any new node can update itself from the network, hence the entire Blockchain, from finance, e-healthcare, public utilities, asset management and government regulations to real estate, logistics and supply chain management. Blockchain has covered a wide range of markets in recent years. Because of its capacity to operate securely without the need for a trusting authority, its enormous success is mainly due. Recent emphasis has been given to a blockchain-based IoMT (Internet of Medical Things) since it not only improves care quality through real-time and continuous monitoring, it also reduces costs (Fig. 11.2).

A growing number of IoMT entities, including sensor nodes, wearable medical devices, patients, hospitals, and insurance companies, are being incorporated into the system. Remote and rapid measurements of vital health indicators, including

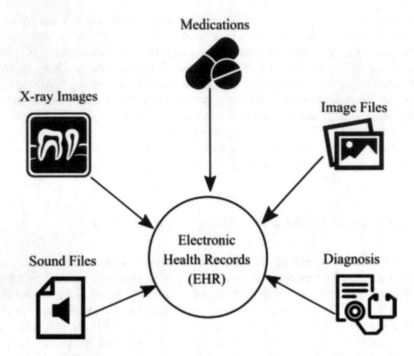

Fig. 11.2 Types of electronic health records

heart rate, temperature, and oxygen saturation, can be made by a doctor using various sensors implanted in or attached to a patient's body. Perception, network, middleware, application, and business make up the first four layers of the IoMT structure, whereas perception, network, middleware, and application make up the final five layers of the IoMT structure. An IoT healthcare system can be used to improve clinical treatment and provide physical and physiological help for patients. The real-time monitoring provided by an IoMT system enhances the quality of care while lowering the overall cost. Accordingly, the IoMT market has expanded from 42 billion $ in 2016 to a projected 150 billion $ in 2021 [17, 18], owing to the escalating expenses of medication and medical device development. Sensors and wearables with wireless connectivity are now talking with a central device, known as a gateway, which typically transmits the received data to the cloud. Wearables, mobile devices, sensors, and other IoMT end nodes deliver real-time data to a cloud-based gateway, and the gateway then determines whether or not to upload the received data into the cloud. Users, including patients, doctors, and healthcare applications, can monitor the end nodes online thanks to cloud-based data. The data that is kept in the cloud can be accessed by users at any time and from any location. IoMT systems must meet a number of requirements, including mutual authentication, scalability, availability, access control and auditability of data, when using a cloud architecture. IoMT application-specific requirements may influence the design process. There are various issues with using a cloud-based IoMT system, such as the availability of services, user privacy and data manipulation. IoMT applications may benefit from the distributed ledger technology of the Blockchain. One of the key advantages of blockchain technology is its distributed architecture, which can alleviate a fundamental problem, namely the cloud's single point of failure in IoMT systems. Additional advantages include smart contracts, data access management, tamper-proof recording and transparency, trustless consensus, and an open architecture that can be used by anybody, regardless of their background. Although this technology has many advantages, it also has several drawbacks, including a lack of standards and regulations, scalability, firmware and hardware vulnerabilities, a lack of trusted authorities and data feeds, and issues with smart contracts like time-stamp dependence, transaction order dependence, and call stack depth. In addition to preserving privacy, blockchain technology has the ability to provide a layer of security that can guard against theft and other hazards. The cloud, on the other hand, offers advantages in terms of network scalability and preventing blockchain forks. Additional considerations include scalability, adaptability and latency in Blockchain-based systems as well as cost considerations and power usage. When using blockchain-based IoMT applications, it is critical to emphasise that patients' medical data must be transmitted and received on time, particularly in remote health monitoring applications such as emergency healthcare and wireless capsule endoscopy. Health information on patients has to be transmitted quickly so that doctors, nurses, and other medical personnel can keep track of them in real-time and provide an accurate diagnosis.

To this day, the vast majority of IoMT systems rely on centralised cloud servers for communication and control. Small-scale IoT networks can now be built using this approach, which has already been used to connect general-purpose computing equipment. The centralised communication approach, on the other hand, cannot keep up with the growing demand for large IoT systems. An IoMT system can benefit greatly from the use of blockchain technology. Using Blockchain, for example, individuals are not compelled to hand over data generated by their IoMT devices to centralised companies. A peer (a node of the blockchain network that has its own copy of the chain) can store data securely, and the Blockchain can verify their authenticity and prohibit unauthorised access.

As a result of the massive expansion in the quantity of personal health records (PHRs) and the subsequent Blockchain, its mechanism has a storage issue. The patient's reports can be uploaded to a distributed ledger, and later doctors or caretakers will be able to monitor those reports remotely from a computer or smartphone. An approved doctor or carer can also view the real-time data received by body sensors. The PHR system could be viewed as a promising solution for the PHR owners' preventive care. The PHR system allows for the transmission of information between healthcare providers and can help predict health problems. Health-related personal data is stored in a personal health record (PHR), which is typically very confidential. Any erroneous tampering with PHR data can have disastrous results that cannot be undone. As a result, every PHR system must-have features that protect user privacy. The most critical characteristic of the PHR system is its tamper resistance. If an individual's lifelong health information can be gathered and saved on

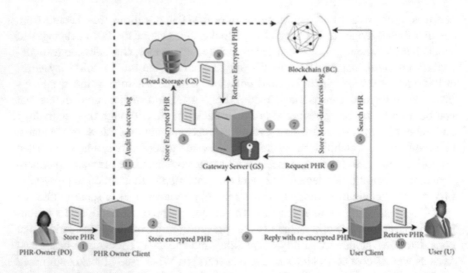

Fig. 11.3 Flow of EHR in smart healthcare systems

tamper-resistant storage, a PHR system can considerably improve the quality of preventive personal healthcare. As a tamper-resistant storage mechanism for PHR systems, Blockchain's immutability, cryptographic verifiability, and back-up capabilities make it an attractive option. Medical records in digital form are called "electronic health records," or "EHRs." Data breaches, security lapses, and privacy violations are all common occurrences when electronic health records (EHRs) are shared among healthcare providers. But with regard to distributed and decentralised communication among nodes in a network (Fig. 11.3).

Blockchain is the twentieth-century technology that provides a distributed and decentralised setting for communication between them without a central authority. A safe, secure, and decentralised environment for exchanging EHR data can be provided by this technology. Researchers have proposed three types of blockchain-based EHR solutions: conceptual, prototype, and implemented. In Blockchain-based IoMT systems, access control is almost regarded in addition to security and privacy, which are the most important elements. Proxy re-encryption used in the access control protocol minimises the need for a gateway server. We can consider the gateway server to be a semi-trusted entity for the sake of this scenario. In order to access the ciphertext of the encrypted PHR data, a group of approved users must be added to the access list. Removing a user's access to their personal health record data is as simple as changing the access list. It is also possible for the PHR owner's delegates to contribute additional PHR data and metadata. The gateway server's local database holds the access control list. The matching secret keys, on the other hand, are guarded by the PHR owner, who owns the secret key. The PHR owner is the only one who can generate the encryption keys used by the gateway server. It is also important to note that the re-encryption keys can only be used by an authorised user to decrypt the ciphertext. Because the actual PHR data is never encrypted at the gateway server, the gateway server cannot access the actual PHR data.

In the healthcare industry, special issues must be addressed when implementing blockchain technology because of its current limitations and potential future scope. The lack of qualified personnel is a major obstacle to medical facilities implementing this cutting-edge technology. There is still a lot of work to be done in the investigation and research of blockchain technology. However, medical societies and regulators must adhere to their responsibilities. The time has arrived for the health care sector to make significant progress. There is a strong likelihood that the use of blockchain technology in healthcare will continue to grow in the future. As a result of this technological advancement, its applications in healthcare will improve because it helps explain treatment outcomes and progress. It is essential to use blockchain technology to verify transactions and move data. Transactions will be authenticated and registered utilising Blockchain technology in the near future with the approval of the network members. As the cornerstone for a new age of health information exchange, Blockchain will guarantee numerical security via public and private key encryption at the patient level. In the future, this technology might be used to improve the security of patient records, prevent infringement, increase interoperability, streamline operations, track medications, and keep tabs on the medical supply chain. In the future, blockchain healthcare is expected to perform exceptionally well.

11.7 Conclusion

Because of its inherent encryption and decentralisation, Blockchain has a variety of useful uses in the healthcare industry. It strengthens the security of patients' electronic medical records, encourages the monetisation of health information, improves interoperability among healthcare organisations, and aids in the fight against counterfeit medicine. One of Blockchain's most important applications is in the healthcare industry, where intelligent contracts can be used to facilitate digital agreements. It is possible to save expenses by eliminating intermediaries from the payment chain with intelligent contracts. There is a strong correlation between Blockchain's potential in healthcare and the adoption of other innovative technologies in the ecosystem. Tracking systems, medical insurance, medicines tracing, and clinical studies are all included. Using device tracking and a Blockchain framework, hospitals can keep track of their services throughout the lifecycle. Patients' medical histories can be better managed with the help of blockchain technology, which can streamline the insurance mediation process and speed up clinical operations. In the long run, this technology has the potential to transform the way patients and doctors interact with and access clinical records, ultimately leading to better healthcare for all.

References

1. Krishna, M & Neelima, M & Mane, Harshali & Matcha, Venu. (2018). Image identification using neural networks. 7. 614. https://doi.org/10.14419/ijet.v7i2.7.10892.
2. Huang, G.-B., Zhu, Q.-Y. & Siew, C.-K. Extreme learning machine: Theory and applications. Neurocomputing 70, 489–501 (2006).
3. Nguyen, G. et al. ML and DL frameworks and libraries for substantial and ample data mining: A survey. Artif. Intell. Rev. 52, 77–124 (2019).
4. Kshitiz, K., et al. "Detecting hate speech and insults on social commentary using nlp and machine learning." International Journal of Engineering Technology Science and Research 4.12 (2017): 279–285.
5. Hitesh Kumar Sharma; Anuj Kumar; Sangeeta Pant; Mangey Ram, "4 Application of Artificial Intelligence in Smart Healthcare," in Artificial Intelligence, Blockchain and IoT for Smart Healthcare , River Publishers, 2022, pp.37–46.
6. Hitesh Kumar Sharma; Anuj Kumar; Sangeeta Pant; Mangey Ram, "5 Application of IoT in Smart Healthcare," in Artificial Intelligence, Blockchain and IoT for Smart Healthcare , River Publishers, 2022, pp.47–56.
7. Hitesh Kumar Sharma; Anuj Kumar; Sangeeta Pant; Mangey Ram, "6 Application of Blockchain in Smart Healthcare," in Artificial Intelligence, Blockchain and IoT for Smart Healthcare, River Publishers, 2022, pp.57–66.
8. Hitesh Kumar Sharma; Anuj Kumar; Sangeeta Pant; Mangey Ram, "7 Security and Privacy challenge in Smart Healthcare and Telemedicine systems," in Artificial Intelligence, Blockchain and IoT for Smart Healthcare , River Publishers, 2022, pp.67–76.
9. Hitesh Kumar Sharma; Anuj Kumar; Sangeeta Pant; Mangey Ram, "8 Electronic Healthcare Record (EHR) Storage using Blockchain for Smart Healthcare," in Artificial Intelligence, Blockchain and IoT for Smart Healthcare, River Publishers, 2022, pp.77–84.
10. Hitesh Kumar Sharma; Anuj Kumar; Sangeeta Pant; Mangey Ram, "9 Methodologies for Improving the Quality of Service and Safety of Smart Healthcare," in Artificial Intelligence, Blockchain and IoT for Smart Healthcare, River Publishers, 2022, pp.85–94.
11. Hitesh Kumar Sharma; Anuj Kumar; Sangeeta Pant; Mangey Ram, "10 Cloud Commuting Platform for Smart Healthcare and Telemedicine," in Artificial Intelligence, Blockchain and IoT for Smart Healthcare , River Publishers, 2022, pp.95–104.
12. Hitesh Kumar Sharma; Anuj Kumar; Sangeeta Pant; Mangey Ram, "11 Smart Healthcare and Telemedicine Systems: Present and Future Applications," in Artificial Intelligence, Blockchain and IoT for Smart Healthcare, River Publishers, 2022, pp.105–116.
13. S. Kumar, S. Dubey and P. Gupta, "Auto-selection and management of dynamic SGA parameters in RDBMS," 2015 2nd International Conference on Computing for Sustainable Global Development (INDIACom), 2015, pp. 1763–1768.
14. Jing Tian, Boglarka Varga, Erika Tatrai, Palya Fanni, Gabor Mark Somfai, William E Smiddy, and Delia Cabrera DeBuc. Performance evaluation of automated segmentation software on optical coherence tomography volume data. Journal of biophotonics, 9(5):478–489, 2016.
15. Ronald Klein and Barbara EK Klein. The prevalence of age-related eye diseases and visual impairment in aging: Current estimates. Investigative ophthalmology & visual science, 54(14), 2013.
16. R. Biswas et al. "A Framework for Automated Database Tuning Using Dynamic SGA Parameters and Basic Operating System Utilities", Database Systems Journal vol. III, no. 4/2012.
17. Sharma, Hitesh KUMAR. "E-COCOMO: the extended cost constructive model for cleanroom software engineering." Database Systems Journal 4.4 (2013): 3–11.
18. M. A. Abadi, P. Barham, E. Brevdo, Z. Chen, C. Citro, for example, is one of the most well-known companies in the world. Using Tensorflow, we can do large-scale machine learning on heterogeneous distributed systems.. preprint arXiv:160304467 arXiv:160304467 arXiv:160304467 arXiv:1603044 (2016).

Chapter 12
Emerging and Digital Technology in Telemedicine System

12.1 Introduction

Telemedicine is the practise of providing patient care and medical education through the transmission of images and sounds using communication and information technologies. The systems that are currently accessible for use in practical telemedicine are changing quickly as new technologies continue to develop.

We think that many medical professionals, including doctors, are aware of the benefits of telemedicine. Scalability is another important consideration because it makes it simple to repeat the communication and invite participation from many additional interested parties located at remote locations, saving us both time and money on physical travel. Telecommunication is still largely unknown in the medical field, while becoming more ubiquitous in the corporate and academic realms.

The rising demand for high-quality images in the medical field is one of the primary causes of this. The finest quality images must be supplied in order to establish accurate diagnoses and offer enough medical information. Additionally, there is a strong demand for moving images to be transmitted in a variety of medical contexts, such as when demonstrating surgery or new techniques. This need creates a significant technical problem because moving images have a far larger file size than still photos, which must be sent smoothly. Tele-radiology, tele-pathology, and tele-ophthalmology are successful examples of telemedicine that use still images, whereas tele-surgery, for example, requires a completely new system to meet doctors' expectations for streaming video. Because telemedicine typically requires specialised equipment, which can be very expensive, cost is a major concern. Hospitals in remote locations and impoverished countries, where telemedicine is most important, might not have the money to buy the required equipment. Due to significant technological improvements over the past 10 years, there are now a number of viable ways for healthcare practitioners to use telemedicine.

S. Gupta et al., *Blockchain for Secure Healthcare Using Internet of Medical Things (IoMT)*, https://doi.org/10.1007/978-3-031-18896-1_12

12.1.1   A Different Healthcare World

The World Health Organization has recently characterized many tasks that digital technology is offering in the area of health, and it is currently developing a set of guidelines for its use in all countries.

These responsibilities include, in brief, providing better and more direct information about health and illness, directly assisting doctors and administrators with patient diagnosis and treatment, offering verifiable and searchable records about births, deaths, and medical encounters, and providing health managers at all levels with operational and strategic information about drug availability, finances, and human resource management. Although we may not fully predict the effects on these functions, it is obvious that there will be upheaval in the manner that healthcare is delivered [1].

12.2   Components of Telemedicine

Due to recent developments in network and wireless technologies, which are linked to recent developments in ubiquitous and nanotechnologies computer systems, the healthcare system has significantly improved over the past 10 years. The use of telecommunications technology for patient care, illness diagnosis, and treatment is referred to as "telemedicine."

This attempts to provide expert-based healthcare, particularly to remote areas with a shortage of staff, through the use of improved communication and telecommunication technologies. Telemedicine, which enables medical treatments to be provided over an electronic network, has transformed the healthcare industry. Teleconsultation, telementoring, and telemonitoring are the three basic subcategories of telemedicine.

12.2.1   Teleconsultation

One of the most well-known subcategories of telemedicine is this one. Fundamentally, it alludes to an online consultation between a patient and a doctor. It can be done by storing a specific image and sending it to the healthcare professional for additional analysis or by using videoconferencing technology.

12.2.2 Telementoring

In this scenario, another who may have more specialized knowledge on how to best assist a patient mentors one medical professional. A good illustration is a doctor who is seeking assistance in managing a patient with autism who lives in a remote area. The best course of action is to connect with a reputable medical organization, which will provide online support from one of their mentors. Telementoring would be that.

12.2.3 Telemonitoring

In this instance, a doctor is connected to a specific biosensor and receives data from a patient who is at home. Any equipment that can properly monitor bio-parameters can be used to perform this task, including an electronic scale, a vital-sign monitor, a glucometer, and others. The doctor will next begin delivering treatment or prescribing medications to the patient based on the test results. With the help of this type of telemedicine, a patient can simply be watched from home without having to visit the medical centre.

12.3 Emerging Technologies in Telemedicine

The healthcare sector has incorporated digital technology, and it is about to change how doctors do their trade. Digital technology has significantly improved operational efficiency in terms of medical care standards. Because of the transformation, both patients and healthcare professionals now have significantly better overall experiences [2].

The increasing use of high-speed telecommunications and COVID-19 have propelled telemedicine and telehealth services into the spotlight. Since the start of the pandemic, the American Medical Association (AMA) estimates that between 70% and 80% of practitioners have started using some kind of this service. Optimizing this sector for use outside of a worldwide pandemic is one of the major issues that still exist. Here is where the application of cutting-edge technologies in telemedicine is useful.

12.3.1   Technologies Proceeding Telemedicine

Worldwide healthcare systems are currently dealing with a perfect storm of both internal and external problems with care delivery. These include overworked physicians, diminishing payments, rising costs associated with providing healthcare, elevated risks to patients and healthcare professionals, and subpar health results. By utilising cutting-edge advancements, the utilisation of smart technology in telemedicine offers the healthcare sector methods to overcome these difficulties.

12.3.2   mRNA Technology

Recently, mRNA technology has gained attention because it is a component of the new Covid-19 vaccinations. Due to their great efficiency, aptitude for rapid development, and potential for low production costs, MRNA vaccines offer an alternative to the traditional vaccine method. A single-stranded RNA molecule called messenger ribonucleic acid, or mRNA, transports the genetic information that is obtained from DNA. mRNA vaccines function by giving cells the genetic information they need to build viral proteins, which the body can then use to mount an immunological defence. The Covid-19 mRNA vaccines' effectiveness has greatly accelerated efforts to create more mRNA vaccines for diseases ranging from cancer to the Zika virus. It is believed that mRNA's promise goes beyond vaccinations. Since almost any protein may be encoded by mRNA, the same fundamental technology might also enable the development of a wide range of treatments by inducing a drug-like reaction in the body [3].

12.3.3   Neurotechnology

Numerous facets of life could be improved by neuro technology. It has many potential future applications in various contexts, such as education, workplace management, national security, and even sports, in addition to the medical and wellness industries, where it is already being used in practice.

All elements created to comprehend the brain, visualize its activities, and even control, fix, or enhance its functioning are included in the field of neuro technology. These components can be created from computers, electrodes, or any other gadget that can be set up to block electric pulses that are passing through the body.

Brain imaging, which captures the magnetic fields produced by electrical activity in the brain, neuro stimulation, which involves stimulating the brain and nervous system to affect brain activity, and neuro devices, an emerging technology that employs an implant to monitor or control brain activity are all examples of how neuro technology is currently used in the healthcare sector. Although most neurodevices are still in the research stage, they have great promise to cure brain problems. Neuralink is a prime instance of this. Neuralink is a device being developed by Elon Musk that will be placed into the human brain to record brain activity and wirelessly send it to a computer. The outcomes of this study might then be applied to electrically stimulate brain activity.

12.3.4   Precision Medicine

Medical technology is becoming more and more individualized to specific people as it develops. Precision medicine takes each patient's unique genetic makeup, environmental factors, and lifestyle into account. For instance, a patient with cancer may receive therapy that is specifically formulated for them based on their particular genetic makeup thanks to precision medicine. As it targets tumours based on the patient's DNA, generating gene alterations and making them more amenable to destruction by the cancer therapy, this personalised medicine is far more effective than other forms of treatment. Great prospects exist for the future of healthcare to be transformed by precision medicine. Precision medicine offers broader, interesting implications beyond oncology, where it is now most advanced, such as in uncommon and hereditary disorders [4].

12.3.5   Clustered Regularly Interspaced Short Palindromic Repeats (CRISPR)

It represents the state-of-the-art in gene editing technology. It functions by utilising the immune system of the invasive viral or bacterial cells. And after that, it can "cut" the DNA strand that is contaminated. The way the disease is handled may alter as a result of this DNA break. Some of our biggest health risks, like cancer and HIV, may be defeated in a few years thanks to gene modification. The potential of CRISPR in the treatment of uncommon disorders is also promising. Cystic fibrosis (CF) is a rare hereditary disease that affects the functioning of the respiratory and digestive systems. The CF gene causes mutations that alter the salt regulation of the entire cell membrane, causing mucus thickening and causing problems in the lungs, pancreas, and other organs. There are several mutations that cause cystic fibrosis, and several clinical trials are currently underway to see if CRISPR can be used to correct these mutations. CRISPR is also being investigated as a possible method for treating sickle cell disease caused by gene mutations. Until recently, bone marrow transplantation was the only real treatment available to patients, but CRISPR gene therapy has given patients new hope. Numerous applications of CRISPR are possible, such as the rectification of genetic flaws, the treatment and advertence of epidemics of illness, and the enhancement of plant growth and resistance. Despite this promise, this technology also poses ethical issues, most notably the human right to "play God" and worries about utilising genetic editing to produce designer offspring.

12.3.6   Health Wearables

Since wearable technology first became popular in recent years—specifically, since the release of Bluetooth in 2000—demand for them has increased. Nowadays, people use wearables that are synchronised with their phones to track a variety of things, including their sleep patterns, heart rate, and physical activity. Wearables can be useful in preventing chronic illnesses like diabetes and cardiovascular disease due to the ageing population in much of the developed world by assisting patients in tracking and enhancing their fitness.

The market for wearable medical devices is still dominated by smartwatches, which are produced by all the big tech companies, including Apple, Google, and Samsung. Depending on the model, they can record electrocardiograms, blood pressure, oxygen saturation, and sleep patterns. Smartwatches with blood glucose sensors are now being developed by manufacturers, which will make it simpler for people with diabetes to manage their condition. Along with smartwatches, other devices such as smart rings, smart garments, and hearables are gaining popularity and are proving to be more and more helpful in gathering data for clinical research.

Technological advancements do not stop with devices worn on the body, insideables and implantable are also in the process of being developed. So far, these microcomputers that work from inside the body have been used to help organs such as the heart and brain function. Insideables, also referred to as smart pills, are considered by many to be the next phase after external wearables. These are swallowed in the form of a hard capsule and send measured values, such as glucose levels, or images from inside the body to aid diagnosis processes. Since implantable and insideables are only just emerging, they are expected to transform healthcare in the years ahead.

12.3.7   Technology in Mental Health

According to estimates, depression will account for the majority of disease burden globally by 2030, necessitating the development of innovative treatments more than ever. Numerous innovative technologies that can assist in addressing patients' continuing mental health requirements have emerged throughout the past year.

Before a patient ever interacts with a clinician, some applications are able to finish patient intake forms and offer an initial diagnosis, and AI-powered technologies are revolutionizing the way mental health treatments are provided. AI Chabot's like Woebot, which can be used in smartphone apps to assist patients practise cognitive behavioural therapy (CBT) techniques, and voice recognition software like Ellipsis can listen for early indicators of emotional distress in a patient's voice and speech patterns. Digital symptom tracking is also essential for improving future mental health services that are effective. Patients are prompted to share data every day by online symptom tracking. An AI programme to spot patterns and notify providers in real time of any danger indications then analyzes the data. Video games are another emerging technology being used for mental wellness. EndeavorRx, which received FDA clearance in 2020, is the first and only video game therapy. The game, which requires a prescription, is meant to help youngsters with ADHD who are 8–12 years old increase their attention span. In clinical studies, 73% of participants said their ability to concentrate attention had improved. Following this accomplishment, video games are expected to become a more widely used, reasonably priced, and easily accessible treatment for a variety of health issues. Recently, it was revealed that DeepWell Digital Therapeutics would establish a first-of-its-kind video game publishing and development company devoted to making games that may amuse players while also delivering, enhancing, and hastening the treatment of a variety of ailments and conditions [5].

12.3.8   Artificial Intelligence

Teleradiology, telepathology, teledermatology, and telepsychiatry are just a few of the telemedicine-related fields where artificial intelligence (AI) is broadening the scope of technology. Intelligent systems powered by AI are making it possible to do more than merely remotely screen patients' diagnostic needs. Examples include care-assistive apps and predictive algorithms. By automatically converting prescriptions into Electronic Health Records (EHRs) and producing medical reports, it lessens the workload placed on healthcare professionals (HCPs), particularly in times of emergency. For instance, Dr. First, a provider of healthcare technology, has unveiled its patented SmartSig AI technology, which accurately enters patient prescription history into hospitals' and health systems' EHRs without the assistance of a person.

HCPs can increase data interoperability and remote patient monitoring with the use of AI-enabled EHRs. Companies like Nuance, 3 M, and Amazon Comprehend Medical are attempting to use this technology with EHR systems. Additionally, AI-based networking models can shorten hospital wait times by accelerating the discovery of specialists. For instance, the Los Angeles County Department of Health Services' physicians decreased the number of visits to specialists by more than 14,000 by introducing telemedicine examinations for diabetic retinopathy at its security net sites.

Healthcare chatbots that use AI are likewise becoming more and more common worldwide. They interact with people virtually, respond to their questions, inform them of sickness signs, and assist in setting up doctor visits. For instance, Engagely AI has created a clever telemedicine bot that collaborates with hospitals to assist them with drug inventory checks, alternative treatment choices, and patient follow-up for regular checkups. Additionally, it enables HCPs to generate digital prescriptions, do remote diagnoses, and verify patient histories.

12.3.9   Augmented and Virtual Reality

All forms of mixed reality (MR), including augmented reality (AR) and virtual reality (VR), and telemedicine work very well together. Clinicians can access real-time data on patients' vitals and experiences thanks to MR technology, which can increase the precision of remote diagnosis.

For instance, the AR startup Iflexion creates apps that support clinicians by providing virtual real-time diagnosis and health monitoring. It fosters effective health management both inside and outside of healthcare institutions and optimises hospital procedures. Medical practitioners can collaborate more effectively on diagnostics with the use of AR-enhanced telemedicine solutions. Clinical experts can share 3D images of their cases with other professionals during virtual consultations using telehealth platforms with AR capability, such as XRHealth.

12.3.10   Tele-robots

Robotics has ventured into a number of telemedicine sectors. Tele-robots facilitate and improve the accuracy of remote patient monitoring, diagnosis, and virtual care. Telerobots can keep an eye on patients' health in real-time and notify doctors if something goes wrong with their condition.

To create robots for remote healthcare environments like ICUs, patient wards, operating and procedure rooms, iRobot has collaborated with InTouch Health. Robots are assisting doctors in scheduling virtual patient visits in addition to remote monitoring. The Florida Hospital, Intermountain Healthcare, and Children's Hospital Boston are just a few healthcare facilities using the two-wheeled robot that VGo Communications developed. It gives physicians who practise from a distance the option to video-call hospitalised patients and get the most recent updates on their health.

The Boston Children's Hospital is also doing a few trial programmes where patients can take telerobots home with them to assist with postoperative consultations and care after their hospital stay.

12.3.11   IoT and Nanotechnology

The Internet of Things (IoT), which focuses on how people, objects, and apps interact with one another, is quickly transforming the healthcare landscape. By providing access to extensive patient data and virtual care networks, it is influencing how technology is used in telemedicine.

Large volumes of physiological and health data, which can be provided by new medical surveillance and diagnostic equipment, are essential for telediagnostics advancements. IoT based on nanotechnology fills this gap. Based on this technology, smart medications and bandages can take photos of the damaged area within the body, gather tissue samples and secretions, and measure body temperature.

A considerably better degree of accuracy in medicine, in terms of both diagnostics and treatments, is finally ensured by the ability to analyse the human body, its medication therapies, and medical devices at the nanoscale. For instance, the Atmo Gas Capsule analyses the gases in the human gut after ingestion and reports any abnormalities. Its sensors can help identify dangerous compounds as well as the body's levels of carbon dioxide and oxygen.

A US-based business called Nanowear has created the SimpleSENSE undergarment and closed-loop machine learning platform, which manages heart failure and allows for remote monitoring. It records and captures phonocardiography, stroke volume, and cardiac output using cloth-based nanosensors. When necessary, this information can be sent to EHR systems to assist doctors with remote evaluations and diagnoses.

12.3.12   3D Printing

It is already possible to create bones, lung tissue, and cartilage using 3D printing in surgery and diagnostic procedures. It is also promising to apply this technology in telemedicine.

A case involving the use of 3D printing for telesurgery has been reported in the New England Journal of Medicine. A splint that was 3D printed straight from the CT scan was used to reconstruct the trachea of a newborn infant. Hearts, bones, and other tissues have also been printed for tele surgeries in the past.

Doctors can print out the contents of remote scans that patients have sent to them using 3D printing. In order to provide an accurate diagnosis and create a treatment plan, doctors can then examine in-depth 3D-printed patient models. Additionally, prosthetics can be 3D printed without the patient being present by prosthetists. We are seeing a growing number of participants, including major tech firms like Amazon, Microsoft, and Facebook, extend their position in this industry as the use of technology in telemedicine grows more widespread. Innovation that prioritizes the requirements of consumers and providers will be crucial for success.

12.3.13   Enhanced Access to Medical Data and Information

Data storage and access has been one of the main advantages of the digital revolution. Patients' data are now accessible to healthcare providers from anywhere. Additionally, the intranet and internet have made it possible for medical practitioners to quickly share medical information with one another, leading to more effective patient care.

12.3.14   Big Data

Digital technology also makes it possible for therapists to quickly collect large amounts of data, which is another huge advantage. Digital technology makes it possible for researchers, clinicians, and those doing epidemiological studies to instantly obtain data from a far more diversified and big population than ever before. Medical personnel may stay up to date on cutting edge practises and trends because to such data collecting, which enables meta-analysis. Additionally, having access to big data enables clinicians to more accurately identify risk factors and suggest suitable preventive or intervention measures.

12.3.15   Improved Lines of Communication

Healthcare personnel to communicate not too long ago once used a beeper. However, today's digital technology has made it incredibly simple for patients and healthcare professionals to communicate. Healthcare professionals can communicate by email, smartphones, text messaging, and other means. Patients no longer need to receive letters in the mail from doctors informing them of their appointments and testing. All of this is now lot simpler and more affordable thanks to technology. Additionally, medical practitioners can use social media, online platforms, and their own webinars and films to communicate with other professionals. It is now simple to converse across geographical boundaries thanks to teleconferencing.

12.3.16   Electronic Health Records

Regarding patient medical records, the advent of digital technology has been a blessing. Large paper files were once transferred from one department to another. During transfer, patient medical charts frequently disappeared or were harmed. In emergency rooms, if patients arrived late at night or on the weekend, it could take a while to locate their medical records. Patients had to be referred through a laborious process, and doctors had to deliver a big package including the medical information. There were many different locations where medical records were kept; some records were still with the internist, some with the psychiatrist, and others with the rehabilitation expert. It was complete anarchy, to put it simply. Electronic health records (EHR), which have made life simpler for both patients and healthcare professionals, have changed all of this. All patient data is now centrally stored and easier to access because to the use of EHRs, which will improve care and produce better results. EHRs also make medical billing quicker, easier, and smoother.

Online learning: The availability of online education, particularly for degrees connected to healthcare, is a key advantage of digital technology. Today, individuals who want to work in healthcare can finish their healthcare degrees entirely online. This gives individuals the freedom to learn when, when, and from whichever school they choose. There is no longer a need for healthcare workers to travel great distances or take time out of work thanks to the availability of online education.

Health Applications: Hundreds of health apps have been created as a result of the digital revolution. With the help of these apps, patients may keep tabs on their health and illnesses, receive medical information, access test results, and receive reminders when it's time for checkups. Additionally, medical professionals can swiftly examine test results, prescription dose recommendations, and other information they urgently require thanks to healthcare applications.

In general, digital technology has changed the healthcare industry. And it is anticipated that this shift will persist in the years to come. The future of healthcare will be altered by innovations like artificial intelligence, machine learning, deep learning, blockchain, wearable technology, and many other similar ones. There is no limit to how far digital technology may advance healthcare as long as organisations serving the healthcare industry and its personnel remain open-minded and develop the necessary infrastructure and systems [6, 7].

12.3.17 Metaverse

There is a heated argument about whether Facebook's switch to Meta and emphasis on shared virtual reality experiences is appropriate. It is ultimately up to you whether or not you are willing to invest in this. Virtual reality in healthcare contexts has considerable promise, even if the metaverse is greatly exaggerated.

Training is one of the most effective uses of VR in healthcare that is currently in use. For doctors, creating virtual training environments can help them hone their abilities and become ready for procedures. VR can also be employed for treatment in particular circumstances. The Virtual Reality Medical Center, for instance, uses VR treatment to assist people with PTSD and phobias like a fear of heights.

12.4 Conclusion

Although there is a growing consensus that digital health will improve the way healthcare is provided in low- and middle-income nations, there are still big obstacles in the way of its adoption and expansion.

We have examined several new telemedicine solutions. All of them are well-liked and promising solutions, but we shouldn't lose sight of the fact that technology is constantly improving, and more practical and affordable systems might be developed at any moment. To fully utilise telemedicine for both healthcare providers and patients around the world, we should keep an eye out for such advances and collaborate closely with engineering professionals.

The power dynamics between the patient and the provider will change as a result of digital technology, altering the responsibilities of both the government and healthcare professionals. However, these shifts will be unavoidable as digital technology becomes more widely used by everyone on the planet. The task of programme administrators and planners will be to make sure that everyone benefits from these developments, not just those who can afford to pay for treatment or have sway over the healthcare industry.

References

1. Kamal Althobaiti. (2021) Surveillance in Next-Generation Personalized Healthcare: Science and Ethics of Data Analytics in Healthcare. The New Bioethics 27:4, pages 295–319.
2. Marc Mitchell & Lena Kan (2019) Digital Technology and the Future of Health Systems, Health Systems & Reform, 5:2, 113–120, DOI: https://doi.org/10.1080/23288604.2019.1583040
3. Shen YT, Chen L, Yue WW, Xu HX. Digital Technology-Based Telemedicine for the COVID-19 Pandemic. Front Med (Lausanne). 2021 Jul 6;8:646506. doi: https://doi.org/10.3389/fmed.2021.646506. PMID: 34295908; PMCID: PMC8289897.
4. Cao MD, Shimizu S, Antoku Y, Torata N, Kudo K, Okamura K, Nakashima N, Tanaka M. Emerging technologies for telemedicine. Korean J Radiol. 2012 Jan-Feb;13 Suppl 1(Suppl 1):S21–30. doi: 10.3348/kjr.2012.13.S1.S21. Epub 2012 Apr 23. Erratum in: Korean J Radiol. 2012 Jul-Aug;13(4):521. Minh, Cao Duc [corrected to Cao, Minh Duc]. PMID: 22563284; PMCID: PMC3341457.
5. Shimizu S, Han HS, Okamura K, Nakashima N, Kitamura Y, Tanaka M. Technologic developments in telemedicine: state-of-the-art academic interactions. Surgery. 2010;147:597–601
6. Anthony B, Jr. Integrating telemedicine to support digital health care for the management of COVID-19 pandemic. Int J Healthc Manage. (2021) 14:280–9. https://doi.org/10.1080/20479700.2020.1870354
7. Matusitz J, Breen G-M. Telemedicine: its effects on health communication. Health Commun. (2007) 21:73–83. https://doi.org/10.1080/10410230701283439

Chapter 13
Artificial Intelligence -Based Cloud Storage for Accessing and Predication

13.1 Introduction

AI is becoming more adept at performing human tasks with more efficiency, speed, and economy. Both robotics and AI have enormous potential in the field of healthcare. Like in our daily lives, our healthcare eco-system is becoming more and more reliant on AI and robotics. The ability to maintain health and reduce the need for medical care is one of AI's most significant potential advantages. Artificial intelligence (AI) consumer health applications and the Internet of Medical Things are already helping people (IoMT) [1]. Technology-related software and apps encourage people to develop healthy behaviours and assist active maintenance of a healthy lifestyle. It gives customers control over their health and wellbeing. AI also improves healthcare professionals' ability to comprehend the everyday routines and needs of the patients they care for, enabling them to better provide feedback, direction, and support for maintaining health. AI is already being used to diagnose diseases like cancer more accurately and earlier. One in every two healthy women who undergo a mammogram receives false-positive results, according to the American Cancer Society.

13.1.1 AI and Machine Learning

The application of AI is making mammography reviews and translations 30 times faster with 99% correctness, which eliminates the need for pointless biopsies [2]. In order to better monitor and identify potentially life-threatening occurrences at earlier, more curable stages, doctors and other caregivers are using AI in combination with the proliferation of patient wearables and other medical devices to manage early-stage heart disease. With the use of cognitive technology, healthcare companies are able to access massive volumes of patient data and enhance diagnosis thanks to IBM's Watson for Health. More medical information than any human can be reviewed and stored by Watson, including every medical journal, symptom, and case study of a treatment's effectiveness ever published. Google's DeepMind Health is working with medical professionals, researchers, and patients to find solutions to real-world healthcare problems [3]. In order to produce neural networks that closely resemble the human brain and incorporate effective general-purpose learning algorithms, the technique integrates systems neuroscience and machine learning. Clinical decision-making and action, as well as administrative task prioritisation, can be aided by predictive analytics. If therapy is to be enhanced, big health data must be used in conjunction with appropriate and timely decisions. The use of pattern recognition to identify those who are at risk of contracting a condition is another area where AI is beginning to take hold in healthcare. AI can help clinicians manage illnesses more holistically, better coordinate care plans, and help patients manage and adhere to their long-term treatment regimens. This goes beyond just looking at medical records to aid in locating patients who are chronically ill and may be at risk of unpleasant episodes. The usage of medical robots dates back more than 30 years. They range from straightforward laboratory robots to highly advanced surgical robots that can operate independently or alongside a human surgeon. In addition to surgery, they have been employed in hospitals and laboratories for laborious tasks, rehabilitation, physical therapy, and support for patients with ongoing issues. Our lifespans are significantly longer than those of earlier generations, and as we get older, diseases like dementia, heart failure, and osteoporosis cause us to pass away more slowly and in a different way. Additionally, it is a stage of life where loneliness is a common problem. Robots could revolutionise end-of-life care by enabling patients to maintain their independence for longer and lowering the demand for inpatient care and nursing facilities. AI is making it possible for robots to go even further and interact socially with humans to keep ageing minds sharp through "conversations" and other social interactions. From research lab to patient, the journey is drawn-out and expensive. The California Biomedical Research Association estimates that it takes a medicine 12 years on average to get from a research lab to a patient. Only five of the 5000 drugs that begin preclinical testing are tested on people, and only one of these five drugs is ever approved for use in humans [4]. Additionally, it costs an organisation on average $359 million to create a new drug from the research lab to the patient. Drug discovery may be one of the most recent uses of AI in healthcare. By using the most recent advancements in AI to automate the drug development and medication repurposing processes, it may be able to significantly cut the time to market for new pharmaceuticals as well as their prices. A trainee's response to questions, decisions, or suggestions might be challenging in a manner that a person cannot due to the development of natural speech and the ability of an AI machine to draw instantaneously from a massive database of scenarios. The challenges can also be continuously changed to match the trainees' learning needs because the training programme can draw knowledge from the trainees' prior responses. Additionally, training can be done on-the-go thanks to the power of AI integrated in smartphones, making it easy to do fast catch-up sessions in the middle of a busy clinic day or while on the road. Cloud computing is now being used more and more in the healthcare industry. The use of cloud computing during the pandemic had been essential to the functioning of the entire healthcare system. Every medical institution, including doctors' offices and hospitals, has benefited from IT infrastructures.

Artificial intelligence and machine learning technologies can assist medical professionals in producing precise medicine solutions that are personalised to the individual characteristics of each patient by processing large amounts of data. It is anticipated that developments in machine learning and artificial intelligence will be of tremendous assistance to clinical investigations involving the central nervous system (AI). In addition to virtual visits and telemedicine, companies that specialise in machine learning are researching and developing methods to streamline processes, as well as strategies to organise and present patient information to clinicians during telemedicine sessions. It is anticipated that artificial intelligence (AI) will have the most significant impact in the field of health care in the twenty-first century. This is because the implementation of artificial intelligence (AI) in the world's healthcare sector will result in enhanced levels of personalisation, product diversity, and affordability, as well as "intelligent" decision-making. The use of artificial intelligence (AI) and machine learning has already begun in a variety of healthcare situations. The versatility of these technologies lends credence to the idea that they could be beneficial in the medical field. AI and machine learning technologies have made it possible for healthcare organisations to use Big Data tools for data analytics, which has enabled advances such as AI-assisted robotic surgery and image analysis. Edge cases are problems or circumstances that can only arise at the very beginning or very end of a range of values for an operating parameter. Finding edge cases is typically required when trying to diagnose rare diseases (the maximum or minimum) [5]. One of the most common applications of machine learning is in the field of medicine, namely in the diagnosis and identification of diseases that would otherwise be difficult or impossible to identify (ML). If you ask anyone who works in the pharmaceutical sector, they will tell you that the process of finding new pharmaceuticals is a difficult and laborious one.

13.1.2 Cloud Computing

It should not come as a surprise that the use of cloud computing is having a significant effect on the medical field. The broad usage of cloud computing makes it possible to achieve innovation as well as control over scalability, and it also makes it possible to access medical records in a more timely manner. Everyone absolutely needs to have access to healthcare on a daily basis; yet, what occurs in the event of an epidemic? There are times when the needs of the medical system necessitate scaling up or down depending on the season, whether it be cold and flu or something more serious. This may be necessary in order to meet the demands of the system [6]. Customers who use cloud computing for healthcare can simply expand or decrease the amount of data storage space they have access to thanks to the cloud, depending on the data requirements of their practise. The best course of action is to constantly be ready for any emergency, as it is impossible to predict when one might occur. It is essential for medical personnel to be able to speak with one another, coordinate requests for extra supplies, and monitor the development of the emergency situation. The use of cloud computing in healthcare has the potential to save lives by delivering essential information to healthcare providers at crucial times and delivering real-time help to newly trained medical professionals. It is now possible, as a result of the use of cloud computing in the medical field, to obtain an important diagnostic directly from your smartphone. This indicates that it is possible to speak with other people regardless of how far apart you are as long as you have access to the internet.

13.1.3 Cyber Security/Cloud Security

At first appearance, cloud computing and cybersecurity may seem to be complete opposites of one another. With the first choice, you have the option of storing your data off-site or constructing virtual walls around it in order to protect it at all costs. When you use the cloud, you are placing the responsibility for the safety of your data and financial transactions in the hands of a third party. (Fig. 13.1).

The most effective method for ensuring that one's network is secure is to maintain all relevant information close at hand and to place one's faith in the

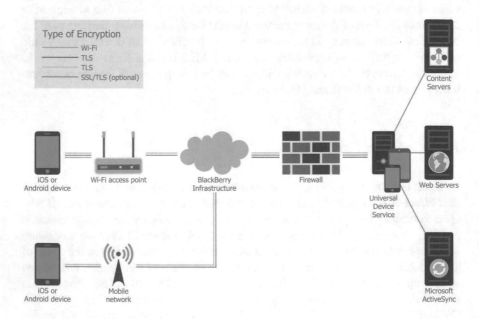

Fig. 13.1 Cloud security architecture

organization's own staff, procedures, and protocols. The medical history of an individual is highly confidential information that must be shielded from any kind of online assault or threat that could arise online. Cloud security is a type of cyber security that is extremely important in this particular scenario. The phrase "cloud security" refers to this type of cyber security.

13.2 Role of Artificial Intelligence, Cloud Computing, and Internet Security in Smart Healthcare

Improved privacy, lower costs, and superior patient care through remote operation and cooperation are some benefits of the rising use of cloud technology in healthcare. The adoption of cloud computing in the healthcare industry opened up new opportunities to improve the efficiency of IT systems. The market for cloud computing is expected to grow at a CAGR of 14.12% from 2022 to 2027 and will reach $71,730.64 million, according to the analysis [7]. Thus, it is clear that healthcare firms embrace new technology and increase their investment in its development. In order to employ remote servers over the internet, cloud computing in healthcare must be implemented. It facilitates the handling, processing, and storage of medical data. Cloud storage makes it simple for medical professionals and institutions to use web servers to safely store a vast amount of data. Such servers are often maintained by IT professionals. Medical businesses have used cloud-based solutions to preserve and secure their patient records in light of the EMR (Electronic Medical Records) Mandate's introduction. Additionally, cloud-based solutions were accepted by healthcare companies even though they had no plans to move their current data centres to the cloud. There has been a significant change in how medical data is produced, used, stored, and shared as a result of cloud computing in the healthcare industry. When it comes to improving data management strategies, the industry has come a long way from the days of conventional storage to the present thanks to the entire digitization of healthcare data. Regardless of the source or location of the data, interoperability focuses on developing data interfaces throughout the whole healthcare system. Through interoperability, healthcare cloud technologies enable seamless sharing of patient information and the gathering of insights to improve healthcare delivery. Healthcare practitioners may now access patient data obtained from many sources, communicate it with important stakeholders, and deliver timely protocols thanks to healthcare cloud computing. Cloud computing and healthcare democratise data and allow patients control over their health. It increases patient involvement in health-related choices and serves as a tool for enhanced patient engagement and education. The fact that medical data may be easily archived and subsequently retrieved when the data is kept in the cloud is another indication of the industry's importance for cloud computing. Data redundancy is drastically reduced as system uptime increases, and data recovery is also made simpler. By granting patients real-time access to medical information, test results, and even doctors' notes, doctors can improve patient involvement with the aid of cloud computing for healthcare. As they gain greater knowledge about their health, this provides the patients power over their health. Furthermore, cloud computing in healthcare prevents patients from being given excessive prescriptions or forced to do pointless tests, both of which can be revealed in the patient's medical data. Collaboration is greatly facilitated by the use of the cloud in the healthcare industry. Patients are no longer need to bring their medical records with them to every doctor appointment thanks to the cloud storage of electronic medical records. The professionals may readily access the data, observe the results of earlier exchanges, and even exchange information in real time. They can then treat patients more precisely as a result. The well-being of the patient is of utmost importance in healthcare, which is becoming more and more dependent on medical systems and technology. The more quickly a patient obtains the proper care in the proper setting with the proper tools, the better the odds of a successful outcome. Patient safety and privacy are also at danger from cyber-attacks on programmes, Personal Identification Information (PII), and Protected Health Information (PHI) [8, 9]. Similar to a ransomware attack, losing access to medical devices and records can encrypt and captive files. Private patient information may be accessed by the hacker and taken. Additionally, the attacker may change patient data mistakenly or on purpose, which could seriously harm the health of the patient. Compliance is essential for the best patient outcomes in the healthcare sector. For sensitive patient information, the Health Insurance Portability and Accountability Act (HIPAA) establishes the bar. To comply with HIPAA, businesses that handle PHI must put in place physical, network, and safety safeguards and make sure that they are followed. Even if there is no PHI breach, failure to do so may result in the imposition of a hefty fee, while a violation may lead to criminal or civil prosecution. The privacy law, security law, notification violation law, and omnibus law are the HIPAA rules' constituent parts. A HIPAA violation could result in a fine for the organisation of $100–50,000 or more.

Among the most important security advice for HIPPA certification is:

- Data security
- Software and network access control layer
- Track violations and restrict access.

Because hackers have access to PHI and other sensitive data, cyberattacks against electronic health records and other systems also represent a risk to patient privacy. Your organisation may be subject to severe fines under the HIPAA Privacy and Security Rules for failing to protect the confidentiality of patient records, in addition to possible harm to its standing in the community. Cyberattacks against electronic health records and other systems pose a risk to patient privacy because hackers can obtain PHI and other sensitive data. For failing to preserve the privacy of patient records, your organisation may be exposed to substantial fines under the HIPAA Privacy and Security Rules, in addition to potential harm to its reputation. For any firm in the medical sector, including healthcare providers, insurers, pharmaceutical, biotechnology, and medical device manufacturers, healthcare cybersecurity is a strategic priority. It entails a range of actions to safeguard companies from internal and external cyber assaults, guarantee the availability of medical services, ensure the proper operation of medical systems and equipment, maintain the security and integrity of patient data, and comply with industry rules.

As a result of advancements made in each of these domains, it is now possible for AI and ML to process extremely large volumes of data with an accuracy that is comparable to that of a human analyst. This was made possible by utilising cloud-based resources, which offer scalability, are more cost-efficient, and provide instantaneous availability. It is becoming increasingly normal practise for healthcare providers at all levels, from primary and secondary care providers to tertiary care specialists, to use data analytics in order to improve patient care. When this information is provided at the moment care is being rendered, it makes it possible for a more accurate diagnosis to be made, which ultimately results in improved outcomes. In both instances, these innovations help bridge the gap between large numbers of patients and a limited number of healthcare practitioners by offering care that is more dependable and delivered in real time. Access to medical treatment is a major issue that needs to be addressed in communities that are spread out geographically. In contrast, digital tools and resources can be provisioned on the cloud and made available over the last mile to these locations that have data network connectivity. This can be done by using the internet. By utilising this technique, primary centres are able to diagnose patients, gather digital samples, and then send those samples on to tertiary centres so that they can undergo additional testing. Tertiary institutions have the ability to quickly access cloud-based data, which enables them to provide cost-effective insights and analyses to their clients. This also enables the preservation of digital data, the analysis of a patient's long-term progression, and the comparison of a group of patients to uncover common treatment courses. Overall, this results in better patient care while simultaneously lowering expenses. Cloud computing makes it possible for machine learning models to become more robust and accurate. Using the cloud's flexible resourcing, it is possible to track extra last mile data from gadgets, wearables, and health trackers, and then stream and aggregate it at a low cost. An infrastructure for computing that is based in the cloud can be utilised to do the heavy-duty analysis of such a large volume of data in an efficient manner. As a consequence of this, the training process will become more effective, and as a result, the accuracy will improve. The scalability of machine learning models improves whenever there is an increase in the amount of data that can be used for training. When it comes to a variety of jobs involving picture processing, for instance, the accuracy of the model has already surpassed that of humans. Customization of machine learning models is possible, which allows for the generation of suggestions that are uniquely suited to meet the requirements of each individual patient. The price of all of this computation is controlled by regulations. Before being used in machine learning models or suggestions, the data relating to a patient need to be encrypted both when they are at rest and when they are in transit and anonymized. This strategy utilises the resources offered by multiple cloud providers and is known as multi-cloud computing. The National Digital Health Blueprint requires strict adherence to privacy and data protection requirements as a prerequisite for implementation [10]. As a direct consequence of this, the establishment of highly developed technical checkpoints is required in order to forestall the accidental disclosure of patient information. In addition, laws relating to consent need to be strictly implemented so that only medical personnel who have the patient's permission and who do so for a predetermined amount of time can access the patient's medical records. In order to accomplish this, it is vital to have cloud environments that are secure, as well as rigorous controls on the access, processing, and dissemination of data.

13.2.1 Artificial Intelligence and Machine Learning (AIML) in Healthcare Systems

Firstly Artificial Intelligence AI is special kind of intelligence shown by machines that can be helped to improved analysis and sentiments. Machines can learn on their own from their past data and the present information provided to them, make sense of the data and use such to do various tasks which can be useful own their own. Artificial Intelligence has helped in improving the present healthcare systems and has helped many patients relentlessly. AI is being used in radiology and chronic diseases like cancer to develop accurate and effective inventions that will assist treat patients who are afflicted by these conditions and, ideally, find a cure. Compared to conventional methods of analytics and clinical decision-making, AI offers a number of benefits. As training data is understood by AI algorithms, the systems become more accurate. This allows humans to get previously unattainable insights into treatment variability, care processes, diagnostics, and patient outcomes. A lot of conventional approaches are also adopted by AI, which has improved upon them in terms of making clinical judgements. AI algorithm provides more precise computation of the data of the healthcare systems as they understand training data which further helps in developing various diagnostic results, patient monitoring etc. Let us see various examples of Artificial Intelligence in healthcare systems.

13.2.2 Early Cancer Diagnosis

Artificial Intelligence has made the hectic work of pathologists quite efficient. PathAI is one of the best machine learning offering tool which provides pathology a whole another dimension to make accurate diagnosis. It reduces the errors during the cancer diagnosis and provides one with the new techniques to apply during diagnosis. As PathAI increases accuracy, cancer can be diagnosed at a particular stage without turning into a fatal one and thus, saving more number of lives.

13.2.3   Diagnosis of Fatal Blood Diseases

AI has improved the diagnosis of blood related problems and making them treated at an early stage thus decreasing the fatality rate. Since AI helps the machines to learn from their previous records for improved results, scientists had already provided machine with 25,000–30,000 blood samples so that AI can make use of them to identify any harmful entities present in the blood sample [5, 6]. This is a fast method of scanning the blood sample than slow paced manual scanning.

13.2.4   Customer Service Chatbots

Nowadays, many AI based chatbots are available for various healthcare services for the patients. They not only solve various day to day queries of the customers but also provides with the many diagnostic solutions to symptoms provided by the patients. This reduces the workload of expert healthcare workers and thus making them to use this time in other handy tasks. These chatbots provide patients with the advanced solutions making better outcomes for the future.

13.2.5   Managing the Medical Records

Since, machine learning involves the use of data science, AI has made easy handling of the medical records of tons of patients and thus saving the time in data management. Like a needle in haystack, data which is valuable can be lost easily making significant loss to a particular industry.

13.2.6   Dosage Errors

AI has helped many experts healthcare workers to make precise dosage for the patients. We know that how a up and down of the dosage prescribed to the patient can lead to serious health illments. AI helps machines to make the perfect dose which is prescribed by the expert. Therefore, with the help of the AI industries can reduce the error margins of the dosage and thus making more efficient results for the diagnosis.

13.2.7 Robotic Surgeries

It is as clear as crystal that how significant difference is made when a work is done by robotic hands and human hands. AI assisted robots are helping many surgeons in improved surgeries. There are surgeries which exceeds the human capabilities such as open heart surgery. Robotic arms provide more precision, flexibility and control thus making hectic surgeries more efficient and reducing the fatality rate. Surgeries which are helped by robot AI results in better treatment for patients thus making an efficient recovery for them with less pain.

13.3 Cloud Computing in Healthcare Systems

Before learning the use of cloud computing in healthcare systems we need to know about cloud computing first. Cloud computing is basically related with the management of the data on internet or managing the services provided through the internet. In simple words it means using the remote servers to maintain and access the data rather than to rely on the private data centers and local hardrives. It provides more cost efficient environment for data storage. Let us see the use of cloud computing in field of healthcare. The main use of cloud computing is that it further facilitates the various technological uses in healthcare systems such as electric assisted medical records, various patient portals and mobile apps for monitoring health related data and big data analytics etc. It also increases the efficiency of the industry with decreasing the cost. Since, healthcare related information needs to be confidential and easily accessible by healthcare related staff, cloud computing helps in such a situation. Doctors can easily manage the data of large number of patients any time and can be securely shared between other members in real time thus, making it perfect companion for the healthcare related workers. Cloud data is very cost effective as it helds large amount of data effectively and securely. Everyone is quite familiar with the environment that healthcare department works in, meaning how socially and flexibily they work. Cloud computing is thus, a perfect companion for that as it lets one work completely under their command socially. Not only that cloud helps healthcare department to provide highest quality services more frequently.

13.4 Security Challenge in Smart Healthcare

The ML models absorb the data from each patient's health tracker, which may be found on a mobile phone or wearable device (like a Fitbit), as well as data from insulin monitoring, sleep monitors, and even blood pressure monitors. In order to process data from beginning to finish, it is necessary to connect all of these devices to the cloud. In view of the stringent legislation and privacy standards, data privacy and access must be continuously monitored and regulated. Because of this, it is necessary to use data management systems that are hosted in the cloud. IT departments need to be equipped with comprehensive management frameworks that can combine corporate and personal devices and carry out the necessary controls in order to safeguard the information they store. Modern unified management frameworks may incorporate the essential governance best practises to control the consumer devices and mobile apps as well as the back end cloud platforms. This will make the situation easier to manage and will make it more palatable for everyone involved.

Healthcare is one of the most weak ventures with regards to network protection. The healthcare framework all over the planet has become more vulnerable to digital assaults in the period of COVID-19. Numerous digital protection associations are detailing a quick expansion in digital assaults starting from the beginning of the COVID-19 pandemic. The healthcare framework, including nursing home, has forever been one of the critical objective of cyberattacks. Late series of assaults in a few significant emergency clinics and healthcare frameworks, have uncovered the security weaknesses of most confided in healthcare organizations. The healthcare businesses are at bleeding edge of worldwide endeavors to battle the infection (COVID-19) during the pandemic. Thusly, this basic area ought to be secure by cybercriminals, yet that isn't what has occurred. The COVID-19 time is portrayed by a precarious ascent in digital assaults, from various culprits and for various inspirations, and the healthcare area has not been secure. The brilliant wellbeing pipeline for information handling and security examination utilizing AI is displayed in Fig. 13.2.

The ideas introduced in this study are based on the ongoing utilization of AI-based advancements, which might restrict our understanding of the maximum capacity of future advancements. Through a survey of the writing and real-world utilizations of AI frameworks in healthcare associations, this study has given a few bearings to successful use and management of AI. We trust our review will animate more thorough hypothetical and exact exploration for the best use of AI frameworks to guarantee the most ideal consideration to patients and give preventive general wellbeing.

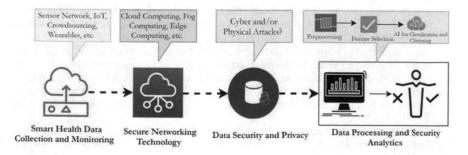

Fig. 13.2 Data flow block diagram for network security

13.5   Conclusion

This chapter describe the present status of man-made brainpower (AI)- based technology applications and their effect on the healthcare industry. Notwithstanding a careful survey of the writing, this study broke down a few real-world instances of AI applications in healthcare. The outcomes show that significant emergency clinics are, as of now, utilizing AI-empowered frameworks to expand clinical staff in persistent finding and treatment exercises for a great many sicknesses. Furthermore, AI frameworks are having an effect on working on the proficiency of nursing and administrative exercises of medical clinics. While AI is being embraced emphatically by healthcare suppliers, its applications give both the idealistic point of view (new opportunities) and the tragic view (challenges to survive). We examine the details of those opportunities and challenges to give a decent perspective on the worth of AI applications in healthcare. Obviously fast advances of AI and related innovations will assist with caring suppliers make new incentive for their patients and work on the productivity of their functional cycles. By the by, powerful utilizations of AI will require compelling preparation and procedures to change the whole consideration administration and tasks to receive the rewards of what advancements offer.

References

1. M. A. Abadi, P. Barham, E. Brevdo, Z. Chen, C. Citro, for example, is one of the most well-known companies in the world. Using Tensorflow, we can do large-scale machine learning on heterogeneous distributed systems. preprint arXiv:160304467 arXiv:160304467 arXiv:160304467 arXiv:1603044 (2016).
2. Krishna, M & Neelima, M & Mane, Harshali & Matcha, Venu. (2018). Image identification using neural networks. 7. 614. https://doi.org/10.14419/ijet.v7i2.7.10892.
3. Huang, G.-B., Zhu, Q.-Y. & Siew, C.-K. Extreme learning machine: Theory and applications. *Neurocomputing* **70**, 489–501 (2006).
4. Nguyen, G. *et al.* ML and DL frameworks and libraries for substantial and ample data mining: A survey. *Artif. Intell. Rev.* **52**, 77–124 (2019).
5. Kshitiz, K., et al. "Detecting hate speech and insults on social commentary using nlp and machine learning." International Journal of Engineering Technology Science and Research 4.12 (2017): 279–285.
6. S. Kumar, S. Dubey and P. Gupta, "Auto-selection and management of dynamic SGA parameters in RDBMS," *2015 2nd International Conference on Computing for Sustainable Global Development (INDIACom)*, 2015, pp. 1763–1768.
7. Jing Tian, Boglarka Varga, Erika Tatrai, Palya Fanni, Gabor Mark Somfai, William E Smiddy, and Delia Cabrera DeBuc. Performance evaluation of automated segmentation software on optical coherence tomography volume data. Journal of biophotonics, 9(5):478–489, 2016.
8. Ronald Klein and Barbara EK Klein. The prevalence of age-related eye diseases and visual impairment in aging: Current estimates. Investigative ophthalmology & visual science, 54(14), 2013.
9. R. Biswas et al. "A Framework for Automated Database Tuning Using Dynamic SGA Parameters and Basic Operating System Utilities", Database Systems Journal vol. III, no. 4/2012.
10. Sharma, Hitesh KUMAR. "E-COCOMO: the extended cost constructive model for cleanroom software engineering." Database Systems Journal 4.4 (2013): 3–11.

Chapter 14
Machine Learning for predictive analytics in Smart health and Virtual care

14.1 Introduction

In the last decade, Artificial Intelligence (AI) has influenced every business, but the progress of AI in the health sector has been gradual [1–3]. Every nation's healthcare system is built and complies with the scenario, weather factors, medical needs of the population, and quality of life in that territory. The dispersion of clinical protocols, tools, medical procedures, therapies, technology, and patient data records across all areas makes automation of the healthcare processing system unfeasible. Using IoT equipment's Intensive Care Units (ICUs), Electrocardiography (ECGs), Magnetic Resonance Imaging (MRIs), and numerous other procedures, electronic health records are captured and stored as extensive databases in either organized or unorganized forms using cloud storage [4–7]. However, not all the data is used for research purposes, resulting in a shortfall of recorded information. Furthermore, most hospitals continue to use conventional methods for patient care, in which patients must travel to the hospitals when they are unwell, wait in lengthy lines in the Outpatient Department (OPD) to see the doctor, and the doctor examines the patient's health. The pharmaceutical method is advised based on the talk, their health expertise, and experience. Organizations must create apps that can be used in the health sector to handle patient information more efficiently and forecast results accurately. The design process, continuing to develop, and deploying such apps is the latest requirement. As a result, organizations have been putting in a lot of effort to use AI to accomplish the goal of creating such apps, which involve the digitization of expansion and modernization of public health care source information and are known as Enterprise Resource Planning Systems (ERP) [8, 9].

ML algorithms have become one of the essential targets by which the healthcare business has gained unique knowledge. Storage capacity has increased over time, allowing it to address critical issues and provide healthcare IT services. This solution-oriented technique is at the heart of healthcare organizations' effectiveness. They've helped to improve the overall attractiveness of the place by bringing across disparate elements. They've also been able to improve the strategy itself by employing crucial domain technology [10].

According to Frost & Sullivan's investigation, AI healthcare will expand by around 40% by 2021 [11, 12]. The data storage industry has seen the most demand for this technology. With the emergence of AI, ML, Natural Language Processing, and Blockchain, data storage has become a simpler procedure. It has taken over as one of the more fundamental methods of gathering sensitive information. More input collected back into the system increases the likelihood of better discoveries and healthier total output. Storage capacity is one of the most crucial parts of the data analytics workflow [13].

14.1.1   Capturing Storage Techniques for Healthcare Data

The emergence of digital technologies is assisting hospitals and health systems in managing their facilities, improving patient care, and controlling expenses. With this inflow of collected data comes significant levels of authority for healthcare IT staff to maintain health records adequately and compliantly. Healthcare businesses are rethinking their backup and recovery systems to meet the growth of data levels to offer unique solutions and apps that regulate privacy and security by the latest healthcare legislation [14–17].

14.1.2   About Healthcare Data

Any data "relating to health issues, fertility results, causes of mortality, and life quality" for a person or community is different health problem information. Clinical measures as well as ecological, economic, and behavioral characteristics are included in healthcare information. Figure 14.1 depicts the key roles of healthcare data storage [18].

14.1.3   Data Storage

When it comes to handling health records, healthcare organizations have three primary options [19]:

- Onsite data storage.
- Public cloud data storage.
- Hybrid cloud data storage solution.

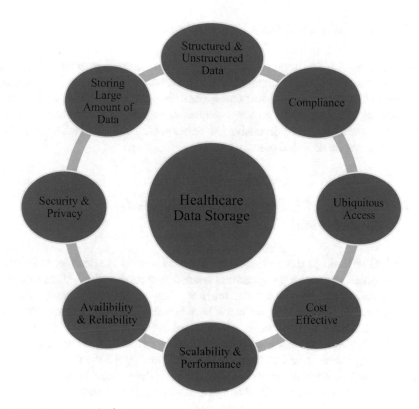

Fig. 14.1 Key roles of healthcare data storage

14.1.4   Onsite Data Storage

For increased control over stored information, health care providers and hospitals choose on-premises storage capacity to securely store patient records. Most health services like the concept of being able to gather information at any time in a secure; local data center, making onsite storage space a preferred option.

14.1.5   Public Cloud Data Storage

The process of sending patient data may be streamlined using cloud-based storage space, making it quick and relatively convenient without sacrificing safety. Cloud computing is more versatile, requiring less money to develop and maintain. Data processing is also much improved. Healthcare firms might begin with a lower amount of cloud space and gradually grow it as the number of data increases [20].

14.1.6   Hybrid Cloud Data Storage Solution

A hybrid cloud-based system combines on-premises storage with public cloud storage as well as the services required to transfer data and coordinate applications between both environments. Most enterprises choose hybrid information storage when scaling up or installing a more complex storage system. Organizations may opt to keep more bandwidth-intensive information on a database machine, such as photos, so it can be accessed quickly [21–23].

14.1.7   Benefits of Storing Data on the Cloud from Multiple Sources

ML and AI will aid in the optimization of diagnostics in the healthcare industry. Patient data that has been aggregated and anonymized can be utilized for prediction, illness modeling, and therapy outcome enhancement. An in-depth examination may reveal patterns for future study, the creation of new medications, or alternative diagnostic procedures. For many firms, cloud-based health data storage makes sense. Integrating health data makes it easier for facilities to maintain test findings and network components to aid in management and therapy. Medical datasets paired with increased processing power will aid in healthcare research and innovation, according to the market. Individual businesses will have more control over the pricing and security of the information migration [24].

14.2   ML-Enabled Storage Systems

In the current era, practitioners are increasingly responsible for gaining patient permission as well as managing health data. Patients' rights to examine, analyze, and trade health data have changed considerably [25]. Despite providing self-tracking information, the majority of people are unsatisfied with their healthcare practitioners. By combining patient healthcare information into contemporary healthcare record systems, it is still feasible to improve patient health care. Various types of patient health information have been recognized in the literature. These categories include prescriptions, demographics, behavioral data, socializing information, genomics, psychology data, disease data, and summaries. To protect the confidentiality of patient health information, a blockchain-based interplanetary file system for secondary storage of health data has been created. Despite this, relatively research has looked into how patients' health data is stored. Securing the patient's confidentiality of information while ensuring data is accessible to important stakeholders is a critical component of good health data management. According to research, health data security is a major concern. The growth of medical gadgets with limited memory and power, as well as large medical data archives, demonstrates this. Many different sorts of organizations are in charge of managing huge amounts of health records [26].

Health data is frequently described as confidential to all individuals, with the same level of protection and anonymity. However, this is not true in actuality since it is not relatively susceptible to being leaked at the same time. Whenever a patient achieves a high level of public recognition, they may provide their cardiologist with the ECG data they obtained on their own. Other healthcare practitioners can access this data via a digital healthcare record. If a patient prefers to keep her maternity test results secret, she may be required to allow her provider to hold them. The sharing of health data among numerous providers that maintain data repositories now allows the storing medium to be suited to the requirements of the patient. Every information chunk's cost, storage, protection, secrecy, and protection are all considered. Heterogeneous implementation approaches, such as the authors', allow confidential information to be stored in cloud storage while no critical data is kept in a cloud environment [27–29]. Nonetheless, it makes no mention of healthcare information analytics. Communication between the two cloud platforms requires time as well, and calculations that rely on speed consume a significant amount of resources. To address this issue, a hybrid cloud platform was created. Medical sensors, applications, and gadgets feed data to AI, allowing for the autonomous detection of medical disorders. Algorithms may classify healthcare information such as ECG, blood pressure, and pulse rate as malignant or benign depending on a variety of parameters and criteria defined by healthcare practitioners [30].

Typical data is frequently useful in clinical research and clinical treatment. An agent-based system was created for older people to save aberrant data using the Body Area Sensor Network. A diversified storage solution is required because health records are created in massive amounts nowadays. Several academics have investigated the profit and quality factors of various Cloud Service Providers (CSPs) to develop strategies for selecting appropriate CSPs for retaining customers' data. Considerable-performance public cloud services save operational time but come at a high cost. Furthermore, academics are looking at blockchain-based techniques for their potential for confidentiality and anonymity in the handling of health information. It is feasible to combine blockchain-based healthcare with conventional medical records, which may be organized depending on user preferences and the potential of using the data in the future. However, because of the way blockchains are designed, they are not suitable for holding vast volumes of health records. Inside the program is a software agent that is familiar with the patient's preferences. Nonetheless, they never provided a method for making this decision. To aid in the selection of store repositories but also elements such as data confidentiality, privacy, and performance quality. Table 14.1 lists the various cloud service providers.

Table 14.1 Different cloud storage platforms [31]

Types and reference	Vendors	Components/ platforms	Purpose	Advantages	Disadvantages	Application
Big data Storage	Google Microsoft Amazon IBM	Cloud Services Azure S3 SmartCloud	The main purpose of is for saving large data and making easily accessible	Enables the allocation of EHRs between certified physicians and hospitals in numerous geographical areas, providing further appropriate contact to life- saving information and falling the need for replica testing	1. Internet bandwidth can be constraint if the speed is low. It may take longer time to upload files and retrieve them 2. If no internet, then no access to the storage 3. Data security and privacy is still a concern	Cloud deployments for clinical applications with isolated or hybrid clouds provided these uses get maximum level of security, privacy, and availability. Nonclinical applications are a better fit for public arrangements but still must be wisely assessed
Relational Databases	Google Microsoft Amazon Cloudera IBM	Cloud SQL Azure MySQL or Oracle MySQL, Oracle, PostgreSQL *dashDB*	They are fully succeeded SQL database service that makes it comfortable to set-up, maintain, bring about and administer relational MySQL databases in the cloud	Can access a familiar, highly available SQL database from MapReduce applications, without having to worry about provisioning, management, and integration with other services	There are connection, size, and app engine specific limits in place	Applications successively on Google app engine or Google compute engine
NoSQL (not only SQL) database [7, 39, 49]	Google Microsoft Amazon Cloudera IBM	AppEngine Datastore Table storage DynamoDB Apache Accumulo *DB2*	Speedy and elastic NoSQL database facilitates for all application need reliable, single-digit millisecond potential at any scale	1. Flexible data models offered by NoSQL databases allow unstructured or semi- structured data to be stored easily 2. NoSQL databases are based on horizontal scalability which allows easy and automatic scaling	1. NoSQL database experts are difficult to get since the application itself is relatively new 2. Though it is claimed that less administration is required, but they still require significant level of skill and effort to install and maintain	Since the significance of EHR application for stability of care and complete health systems, using NoSQL databases have important possible to lead to superior EHR applications in terms of scaling, flexibility and greater obtainability

14.3 The Current State of Technology

In the backup and recovery arena, there is a more substantial difficulty in terms of security. While safeguards are now being implemented, relatively few of them address the greater backup and recovery paradigm. When it comes to understanding security, having the appropriate methodology is crucial from a data standpoint. Companies may invest in the beneficial long-term preservation of data sets throughout the panel by using essential technologies such as Blockchain and ML. There are further benefits to employing predictive modeling in the industry, as suppliers are experiencing higher Returns on investment (RoI).

Merck collaborates with Atom Wise to improve its secure data storage using Deep Learning (DL). It's one of the best illustrations of how AI and ML can make data analysis safer. It's also a better technique to assure a digital storage model's lifetime. Organizations like Merck have been able to maintain their success by utilizing advanced technologies and in-depth data. Improving the essential offering results in a more extensive overarching strategy.

Storage capacity is critical, but so is maintaining compliance with all security procedures. It is critical to tackle storage space with a security-first mindset. This will provide stronger overall security and make firms more compliant with all processes. But there is always a risk of a data breach. Businesses must be watchful against such assaults. From a security aspect, the healthcare industry must take the appropriate precautions to avoid theft.

There is an inherent problem with storage devices that focuses on the system's security. If the process is open and there are numerous stakeholders engaged, the data might be stolen from outside sources. There is also the possibility of manipulation during the storage procedure, as well as difficulties that may occur from external validation. There may also be instances where contributions from outside the industry damage the entire data storage procedure. For improved healthcare, the business must maintain its safeguards and establish a more compliant atmosphere.

14.4 Enhancing Existing Enterprise Data Warehouses (EDW)

It is critical in healthcare to have the correct digital storage systems that operate well with EDW. This is crucial to maintain since interoperability is critical, particularly when dealing with decades-old data warehouses. This is also vital to completely investigate because there have been occasions when the data has been proved to be inaccurate, resulting in inconsistencies in outcomes when there is poor integration. The EDW must be scalable and integrated with the present tools being used. As a result, digital storage techniques must be employed to improve EDW platforms [32].

Backup and recovery tools must also enable accessibility across the enterprise. There should be no scenarios in which more data is provided than is necessary. In certain circumstances, metadata is transferred across a protected network, which breaches regulatory requirements. As a result, the data storage technologies employed must be scalable and dependable enough to provide correct adherence and privacy.

Backup and recovery tools are extremely important from the standpoint of research laboratories all around the world. The equipment you use will influence your study project in more ways than one. It may also help to outline its overall strategy and make the organization quite compatible with industry best practices. When the proper backup and recovery tools are used, there are no issues with performance evaluations or statistics. For experts, this is where the variety of experiences intersects, and they can completely rely on the findings. This is one of the largest contributors to the global health industry. As governments improve their data collection capabilities, they will be able to run better analyses.

14.5   Background Work

When it comes to obtaining the appropriate volume of data, there is indeed a lack of certainty. There is also a lack of consistency in data storage techniques at the moment. Both people and machines are capable of making biases and mistakes. From an outcome standpoint, this involves choices in storage devices. This is when you're seeking the proper information while none is available. This is also where sampling mistakes and standard error issues arise. It produces a lesser end product. It also leads to more uncertainty in the outcomes. This is detrimental to the health sector itself.

Data availability is also a key concern. While data may not be present everywhere, there may be locations where data is not present in sufficient quantities. Sample sizes are too tiny to perform in this case. The data entry employee or analyst may not fully comprehend why they are documenting. This may cause complications as a result of the action. While the difficulty of obtaining quality data persists, there is a greater demand in the sector for improved data storage technologies [33].

There is a greater demand for better data capture systems in the healthcare industry. This is especially true in the AI field, where more data is required to calculate better algorithms. Otherwise, there are flaws in the programming, and the data no longer powers the analytics. The information must be a cogent participant in the digital transformation that is now taking place in the healthcare arena. As a result, businesses and research institutions in healthcare must invest in more data storage solutions.

It is critical to saving better data at the source. This is accomplished via the use of increasingly automated technologies and solutions that are meant to ensure a more integrated approach. This allows businesses to collect more data and provides a more dynamic data center for analytics [34].

The techniques for collecting data grow in tandem with the tools. This results in a more comprehensive approach to data analytics and the incorporation of best practices. Data storage at the source also covers several ways that healthcare providers might employ. Some solutions use the capabilities of Blockchain to make raw data retrieval and storage more secure. This is an effective method of preserving data in your dashboard.

The practical training necessary to optimize usefulness is another important feature of the storage mechanism. When research businesses hire the proper people for a project, they must guarantee that they are using the right technical tools. The core personnel must be informed enough to see the value of the technology being used. Another thing to consider is the scalability of the instrument being utilized. This is vital to evaluate because every healthcare initiative generates a large amount of data. With data, there is a demand for greater scalability, which eventually leads to improved data storage at the source.

In addition, storage capacity is rarely linear. There are several sources to consult, as well as numerous data sets to examine separately. When projects span numerous years, it is critical to have a data storage technology that is cross-domain compatible. It's also more appropriate in terms of scale. When organizations grow in scope, data storage technologies can serve as an integration bridge, storing and analyzing data from many sources. It makes perfect sense from a resource aspect to choose a suitable data storage solution. As research gets more organized, new technologies on the market that integrate with existing healthcare systems emerge [35–37].

14.6   ML Techniques for Treatment of Healthcare Data

The healthcare business has been expanding with the help of artificial intelligence. Massive amounts of data are gathered by IoT devices and thereafter stored on virtualized external platforms. The mix of IoT, big data, and the cloud has proven to be the key to the industry's revolution. The massive amount of data gathered is meaningless unless it is leveraged to generate meaningful findings through the process of knowledge discovery. As a result, data science has incredible possibilities, and efforts are being made to create applications that can use AI and ML to simplify the provision of healthcare resources to the public and assist doctors in using ML techniques in addition to their experience and medical expertise in assessment and treatment [38].

A smart health monitoring system that will deliver a tailored analysis of heart patients' ECG data to forecast the risk of cardiovascular disease. When the parameters influencing the emergence of the disease surpass threshold levels, the physician can use the recommendation system, which employs visualization and classifiers, to alert the doctor. Following the application of several ML models, it is determined that a Support Vector Machine (SVM) is the best choice for the database when the training data is substantial.

PredictT-ML is an analytical software application that predicts outcomes based on clinical data. The goal of the tool development is to streamline the process of feature extraction, methodologies, and hyper-parameter classification, thereby reducing the workload of research scientists who must individually iterate different hyper-parameter values and choose various ML models to improve the system's reliability.

Using real-time hospital data, a Convolutional Neural Network-based Multimodal Disease Prediction (CNN-MDRP) system was developed to predict the probability of cerebral ischemia. The demographic information, behaviors, and illnesses of the patients were saved as structured data, whereas the illness descriptions provided by the patients were stored in unstructured textual formats. Later, k-nearest neighbors (k-NN), decision trees, and SVMs were the ML algorithms used to produce the illness on structured information. The predictive accuracy was 94.8% [39].

A strategy for optimizing the deployment of Virtual Machines (VMs) for the implementation of machine learning algorithms to diagnose and forecast Chronic Kidney Disease (CKD). ML algorithms such as linear regression and Artificial Neural Networks (ANNs) are used to predict the outcome of illness diagnosis. VMs are optimized using Parallel Particle Swarm Optimization (PPSO). Each disease necessitates the development of a model based on the estimation causing the disease, which adds to the idea's future direction.

14.7 Smart Access Techniques for Storage Systems

The accuracy of ML techniques such as SVM, logistic regression, random forest classifier, Gaussian Nave Bayes, and decision tree classifier is compared. With an accuracy of 88.29%, logistic regression fared the best. Various machine learning algorithms may be modified to assess massive patient records held in various digital medical devices used in critical care units, operating rooms, ventilators, and clinics. As a consequence, this data is initially pre-processed utilizing filtering methods before being utilized to apply multiple ML frameworks to predict the correctness of the outcome.

14.8 Prediction of Diseases on Healthcare Data, Both Batch, and Real-Time Data Streams

Health records will gradually be stored in many repositories, allowing patients to choose the repository that best matches their needs. Patients should avoid utilizing a single source for all of their health data since the context of therapy, data trends, and regulatory limitations may change. A selection algorithm must be created to automate the storage decision. This is especially true when it comes to continually flowing health data. Choosing the best repository is a difficult procedure. Regulatory problems must be considered in addition to an understanding of storage characteristics utilized for interoperability, data security, and privacy.

Big data cannot be stored, retrieved, or evaluated using a unified patient records system. When electronic health records fail, patients may lose critical information. Caregivers' reactions were hindered due to the manual transfer of data collected by sensing devices to personal health information. As a result, techniques for storing patient-generated health data on commercial blood glucose monitors were created. If the streaming data is processed or compacted, the electronic health information system can be designed to accommodate it.

Different strategic plans and standards have been proposed to encourage the use of an electronic health record system. Functional needs, troubleshooting, and optimization features should all be considered when choosing an electronic health record. The author presents a checklist of measures to take before purchasing an electronic health record system. Checklists often involve on-site customer meetings, site visits, and the maintenance of live processes. Hospitals, clinics, insurers, and patients should all have their health data connected to centralized systems.

Because of their large volume and frequency, patient-centered health data with high degrees of structural heterogeneity must be saved and processed fast. Precision is necessary for health data to deliver helpful insights; however, some sources generate ambiguous and erroneous information. These challenges can be alleviated by using distributed data storage systems. A variety of cloud storage media has been investigated. To forecast the thermal sensibility voting system, an ML and DL model are employed.

Employing blockchain and Interplanetary File Systems (IPFS), a compression method is used to access health repository data as quickly as possible with no data loss. DL and ML algorithms are used to efficiently classify diabetic retinopathy. Using an Adaptive Genetic Algorithm with Fuzzy Logic (AGAFL), a genetic algorithm with fuzzy logic can assist medical practitioners in diagnosing cardiac problems at an early stage. The selection of repositories did not take into account health database systems or data quality. Additionally, no ML algorithms to respond to user interests were established.

14.9 Conclusion

Storage capacity has been one of the most important ways that the healthcare business has evolved through time. There have been several fields formed inside space as a result of the innovation provided by key technologies. Everything from AI/ML to embedded sensors has been improved by utilizing the appropriate kind of digital storage solutions. Storage capacity has progressed to the point where new technologies are available to capture higher quality and quantity of data. The healthcare corporate data economy has improved due to an increase in the quality of important data. This data can yield insights that are becoming increasingly relevant in the healthcare industry.

References

1. Plastiras P, O'Sullivan D. Exchanging personal health data with electronic health records: A standardized information model for patient-generated health data and observations of daily living. Int J Med Inform. (2018) 120:116–25. https://doi.org/10.1016/j.ijmedinf.2018.10.006
2. Cortez A, Hsia P, Mitchell E, Riehl V, Smith P. Conceptualizing a data infrastructure for the capture, use, and sharing of patient-generated health data in care delivery and research through *2024 (white paper). (2018).
3. Chung CF, Dew K, Cole A, Zia J, Fogarty J, Kientz JA, et al. Boundary negotiating artifacts in personal informatics: Patient-provider collaboration with patient-generated data. In: Proceedings of the 19th ACM Conference on Computer-Supported Cooperative Work & Social Computing, (2016). p. 770–786. https://doi.org/10.1145/2818048.2819926
4. Lordon RJ, Mikles SP, Kneale L, Evans HL, Munson SA, Backonja U, et al. How patient-generated health data and patient-reported outcomes affect patient-clinician relationships: A systematic review. Health Inform J. (2020) 26:2689–706.
5. S. K. Ramakuri, P. Chithaluru, and S. Kumar. "Eyeblink robot control using brain-computer interface for healthcare applications." International Journal of Mobile Devices, Wearable Technology, and Flexible Electronics (IJMDWTFE) 10, no. 2, pp. 38–50, 2019.
6. Albahri A, Zaidan A, Albahri O, Zaidan B, Alsalem M. Real-time fault-tolerant health system: Comprehensive review of healthcare services, opens issues, challenges, and methodological aspects. J Med Syst. (2018) 42:137. https://doi.org/10.1007/s10916-018-0983-9
7. Isern D, Moreno A. A systematic literature review of agents applied in healthcare. J Med Syst. (2016) 40:43. https://doi.org/10.1007/s10916-015-0376-2
8. Vaidehi V, Vardhini M, Yogeshwaran H, Inbasagar G, Bhargavi R, Hemalatha CS. Agent-based health monitoring of elderly people in indoor environments using wireless sensor networks. Procedia Comput Sci. (2013) 19:64–71. https://doi.org/10.1016/j.procs.2013.06.014
9. Ko SY, Jeon K, Morales R. The hybrid model for confidentiality and privacy in cloud computing. HotCloud. (2011) 11:8. https://doi.org/10.5555/2170444.2170452
10. S. Kumar, G. H. Sastry, V. Marriboyina, H. Alshazly, S. A. Idris, M. Verma, and Manjit Kaur. "Semantic Information Extraction from Multi-Corpora Using Deep Learning." Computers, Materials and Continua pp 1–17, 2021.
11. Stranieri A, Balasubramanian V. Remote patient monitoring for healthcare: a big challenge for big data. In Managerial Perspectives on Intelligent Big Data Analytics. IGI Global, (2019). p. 163–179. https://doi.org/10.4018/978-1-5225-7277-0.ch009
12. Ruiz-Alvarez A, Humphrey M. A model and decision procedure for data storage in cloud computing. In Proceedings of the 2012 12th IEEE/ACM International Symposium on Cluster, Cloud and Grid Computing (grid 2012). IEEE Computer Society, (2012). p. 572–579. https://doi.org/10.1109/CCGrid.2012.100
13. Ruiz-Alvarez A, Humphrey M. Toward optimal resource provisioning for cloud MapReduce and hybrid cloud applications. In: Proceedings of the 2014 IEEE/ACM International Symposium on Big Data Computing. IEEE Computer Society, (2014). p. 74–82. https://doi.org/10.1109/BDC.2014.
14. Yoon MS, Kamal AE. Optimal dataset allocation in distributed heterogeneous clouds. In: 2014 IEEE Globecom Workshops (GC Wkshps) IEEE, (2014). p. 75–80. https://doi.org/10.1109/GLOCOMW.2014.7063389
15. Zhang Q, Lu J. Artificial intelligence in recommender systems. Complex Intell Syst. (2021) 7:439–57. https://doi.org/10.1007/s40747-020-00212-w
16. P. Chithaluru, R. Tanwar, and S. Kumar. "Cyber-Attacks and Their Impact on Real Life: What Are Real-Life Cyber-Attacks, How Do They Affect Real Life and What Should We Do About Them?." In Information Security and Optimization, pp. 61–77. Chapman and Hall/CRC, 2020.

17. Stock C, Dias S, Dietrich T, Frahsa A, Keygnaert I. Editorial: How can We Co-Create Solutions in Health Promotion with Users and Stakeholders? Front. Public Health. (2021) 9:773907. https://doi.org/10.3389/fpubh.2021.773907

18. Andy YY, Shen CP, Lin YS, Chen HJ, Chen AC, Cheng LC, et al. Continuous, personalized healthcare integrated platform. In TENCON 2012 IEEE Region 10 Conference. IEEE, (2012). p. 1–6. https://doi.org/10.1109/TENCON.2012.6412226

19. Peleg M, Shahar Y, Quaglini S, Fux A, García-Sáez G, Goldstein A, et al. Mobiguide: a personalized and patient-centric decision-support system and its evaluation in the atrial fibrillation and gestational diabetes domains. User Model User-Adapt Interact. (2017) 27:159–213. https://doi.org/10.1007/s11257-017-9190-5

20. Hohemberger R, da Rosa CE, Pfeifer FR, da Rosa RM, de Souza PS, Lorenzon AF, et al. An approach to mitigate challenges to the electronic health records storage. Measurement. (2020) 154:107424. https://doi.org/10.1016/j.measurement.2019.107424

21. Business NA. How can I choose the best electronic health record system for my practice? Neurology. (2010) 75:S60–4. https://doi.org/10.1212/WNL.0b013e3181fc9888

22. Weathers AL, Esper GJ. How to select and implement an electronic health record in neurology practice. Neurol Clin Pract. (2013) 3:141–8. https://doi.org/10.1212/CPJ.0b013e31828d9fb7

23. Hart EM, Barmby P, LeBauer D, Michonneau F, Mount S, Mulrooney P, et al. Ten simple rules for digital data storage. PLoS Comput. Biol. (2016) 12:10. https://doi.org/10.1371/journal.PCBs.1005097

24. Wilson G, Bryan J, Cranston K, Kitzes J, Nederbragt L, Teal TK. Good enough practices in scientific computing. PLoS Comput Biol. (2017) 13:e1005510. https://doi.org/10.1371/journal.PCBs.1005510

25. Khan SI, Hoque ASML. Towards the development of health data warehouse: Bangladesh perspective. At the 2015 International Conference on Electrical Engineering and Information Communication Technology (ICEEICT). IEEE; (2015). p. 1–6. https://doi.org/10.1109/ICEEICT.2015.7307514

26. Mackey TK, Kuo TT, Gummadi B, Clauson KA, Church G, Grishin D, et al. 'Fit-for-purpose?'–challenges and opportunities for applications of blockchain technology in the future of healthcare. BMC Med. (2019) 17:68. https://doi.org/10.1186/s12916-019-1296-7

27. Rehman SU, Javed AR, Khan MU, Nazar Awan M, Farukh A, Hussien A. PersonalisedComfort: a personalized thermal comfort model to predict thermal sensation votes for smart building residents. Enterpr Inf Syst. (2020). 1852316. https://doi.org/10.1080/17517575.2020.1852316

28. Mubashar A, Asghar K, Javed AR, Rizwan M, Srivastava G, Gadekallu TR. Storage and proximity management for centralized personal health records using an IPFS-based optimization algorithm. J Circ Syst Comput. (2021) 2250010. https://doi.org/10.1142/S0218126622500104

29. Gadekallu TR, Khare N, Bhattacharya S, Singh S, Maddikunta PKR, Srivastava G. (2020). Deep neural networks to predict diabetic retinopathy. J Ambient Intell Human Comput. (2020) 1–14. https://doi.org/10.1007/s12652-020-01963-7

30. Reddy GT, Reddy MPK, Lakshmana K, Rajput DS, Kaluri R, Srivastava G. Hybrid genetic algorithm and a fuzzy logic classifier for heart disease diagnosis. Evol Intell. (2020). 13:185–96.

31. Trojer T, Katt B, Schabetsberger T, Mair R, Breu R. The process of policy authoring of patient-controlled privacy preferences. In: International Conference on Electronic Healthcare. Springer, (2011). p. 97–104. https://doi.org/10.1007/978-3-642-29262-0_14

32. Analytics V. What is confusion matrix (2020). Available online at: https://medium.com/analytics-vidhya/what-is-a-confusion-matrix-d1c0f8feda5 (accessed November 17, 2020).

33. S. Hijazi, A. Page, B. Kantarci, T. Toyota, Machine learning in cardiac health monitoring and decision support. Computer 49(11), 38–48 (2016)

34. G. Luo, PredicT-ML: a tool for automating machine learning model building with big clinical data. Health Inf. Sci. Syst. 4(1), 5 (2016)

35. M. Chen, Y. Hao, K. Hwang, L. Wang, L. Wang, Disease prediction by machine learning over big data from healthcare communities. IEEE Access 5, 8869–8879 (2017)

36. Mandal, Machine learning algorithms for the creation of clinical healthcare enterprise systems. Enter. Inf. Syst. 11(9), 1374–1400 (2017)
37. K. Shameer, K.W. Johnson, B.S. Glicksberg, J.T. Dudley, P.P. Sengupta, Machine learning in cardiovascular medicine: are we there yet? Heart 104(14), 1156–1164 (2018).
38. G. Meyfroidt, F. Güiza, J. Ramon, M. Bruynooghe, Machine learning techniques to examine large patient databases. Best Pract. Res. Clin. Anaesthesiol. 23(1), 127–143 (2009)
39. D. Swain, P. Ballal, V. Dolase, B. Dash, J. Santhappan, An efficient heart disease prediction system using machine learning, in Machine Learning and Information Processing (Springer, Singapore, 2020), pp. 39–50.

Chapter 15
Smart Healthcare and Telemedicine Systems: Present and Future Applications

15.1 Introduction

As there has been a sudden increase or growth in the population getting covid positive and are becoming critically unwell there is a need of improvements in the building of vast amount of hospitals and also the duration of the stay needed to be increased for the welfare of the patient with the help of decreasing the cost for the health care services. Telemedicine used in the ICUs it is basically considered as closing or reducing the gap between the demands and the supplies [1]. It has been seen or observed that there was a vast or great amount of change in the percentage of the number of hospitals from 0.4% to 4.6% from the year 2002 to 2010. As an enhancement or improvement, telemedicine is being used as the addition of the audio-visual conferencing technology to for exchanging of the information for assisting the treatment clinically for the patient in at ill conditions. Nurses for the critical care nurses can access the electronic medical records whose main purpose is to provide the nurse with the patient's details such as lab outputs or outcomes images which have been taken out or generated from the radiographs, information related to the telemetry which helps in the detection of the changes in a patient's condition and at the same time alert them about the same. There have been various improvements in the measures in the field of telemedicine systems such as helping to create a well coherent plan for care with respect to the diseases related to the patients. As the work culture in today's world have rapidly made their growth which has resulted into a greater and as well as higher risk of errors in the medical field. Increased rates of best practices and methods in the field of critical caring has helped in reduction of the deep vein thrombosis. Recent advancements in the fields of telemedicine have brought decision support tools and the smart alarm systems to the tele-ICU technology [2], which allows response on time and recognition of prompts to see changes in the status and health of patients. With the growing rate of artificial intelligence and Machine Learning, there has been an immense rate of increase in the field of ML being used in the field of the telemedicine, which has been used as the source of flow of the data related to the patients continuously which is sensitive to with respect to the conditions of the patients health. Machine Learning with Telemedicine ML algorithms have also been used in the sepsis detection and reducing the alarms causing fault decisions to occur. For the future betterment in the field of telemedicine technology a framework has been planned which can be considered as the business model for generating a regional innovation system, most importantly for the people or population living in rural areas. As healthcare and education can be combined together for an improvement in the education field as well known as the tele-education, in which mobile technologies can be considered along with tele-education for helping students keeping touch with their mentors, with the ongoing placements of the seniors opportunities could be provided. Regional Innovation System (RIS) considers the spread considering a certain or a specific social system [3]. RIS if looked at a wide angle can be used as the knowledge generation and applications and as a diffusion subsystem in the field of telemedicine for an accurately interactive sessions with the known organizations and for conducting interviews in a structured manner for the completeness of their frameworks. There has been an immense effort made in improvement of the telemedicine field with the tele-education systems which can be listed as identification of the agents for development of strategies for overcoming these gaps. The methods for an improved structured manner of conducting interviews are as follows validating and updating the framework interviews held. Different organizations were chosen or selected on the basis of their activeness in the field of telemedicine systems. Teleconference was made for taking a grouped discussion on what have been the improvements that can be brought into the present or the current telemedicine system. AS far as cloud technologies are being concerned they have also been used or contributed to the field of the telemedicine and tele education systems (Fig. 15.1).

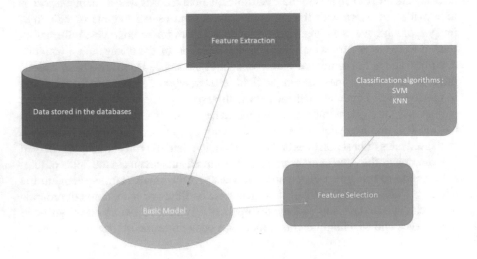

Fig. 15.1 Voice impairment for Parkinson's disease using machine learning

15.2 Smart Healthcare Tools and Techniques

Smart healthcare can only be made through the collaboration of different IT sectors among which we'll discuss Artificial Intelligence, Blockchain, Internet of Things, Cloud Computing. All these above-mentioned domains need to support each other to make the system work properly. These are some of the most dominant domains of the industry and needs the work of professionals only. As we are creating a healthcare system which will work towards the well-being of a person, we can't show any carelessness. Telemedicine system a system in which the doctor can check on the patient remotely or they don't need to be in the same room. This type of system could've been very efficient in the COVID-19 pandemic time because the doctor can check on the patient without making any physical contact at all. This would've helped in significantly providing help to patients as well as decreased number of doctor's would've been affected by COVID-19 from doing check-up of the patients [4]. Now let's take a look at the use of artificial intelligence in making this system and software. The AI is the most important component in the making of every digital thing. Artificial intelligence would be used in the smart healthcare system to help manage the system more efficiently like it could redirect the user to the required article or anything that the user has searched for. It can very well give out proper instructions if a user is having a problem in using the system.

AI will be responsible for helping the doctors and patients in the telemedicine system. A doctor can view the results data faster and in the desired sorted way because the AI will do it according to the doctor's need and will help in making the session with the patient more to the point. The AI can also remind the patient of the doctor's prescription from time to time, which will help to avoid any type of delay the patient might have suffered if he forgets to take the medicine on time. Let's look at the role of blockchain now, it helps to safely store and retrieve the data. It'll be used to store the data of the patient and it gives fast retrieve speed which will help anyone in finding it quickly through proper means. Blockchain is popular only because it offers security in storing the files and makes it harder for an interference to find it. In the smart healthcare system, it'll be blockchain that would store the immediate data of the patient or the user and will ensure that it gets sent to the other side safely. Now comes IoT or Internet of Things, it'll help in retrieving the data from the health device and will connect it to the other device with the help of blockchain. We've discussed in the previous assignment that how IoT devices are great and how blockchain helps to mitigate the security issues that IoT creates. Without the help of IoT devices it won't be possible to make the telemedicine system because there won't be any device that would automatically record the required health stats of the patient that the doctor or health consultant would require to give the prescription. IoT is necessary to connect the required devices to the network so that the formed network can perform properly in solving the issues it is supposed to solve. It is a huge asset to the industry that making use of IoT is not a very tough task. It is simple to apply but hard to keep safe from other interferences. Let's talk about cloud computing, it is necessary to save all the records of all the patients for future reference or research. This huge amount of data is stored with the help of cloud computing, it helps by storing large amount of data that the system and organisations require to function properly. Cloud storage is different from blockchain because unlike blockchain which stores data at different places forming blocks, cloud on the other hand stores the data at server at a different place. This is also the reason that cloud is used for storing large amount of data that will be required at a later date whereas blockchain mainly stores data for immediate use with strong transfer safety. Talking about the healthcare system as a whole we realize that it'll be very helpful in the present and the future. The healthcare system in the present would be good enough for the basic check-ups as well as accessing information regarding medical issues. It'll take time for people to adjust to it as it'll be the first of its type with so many features. The healthcare system would be effective in the future as well and by that time people would be used to it. It'll get a lot of quality-of-life updates making it more effective at its job. It will use a smarter AI and an enhanced IoT device [5].

15.2.1   Cloud Computing in Smart Healthcare

When it comes to talking about the various models of the cloud computing, there are mainly two of them which are deployment model and the other being the service model. This has been represented with the help of a flow diagram for the same: (Fig. 15.2)

The deployment model further consists of three major types that are listed below:

- Public Cloud
- Private Cloud
- Hybrid Cloud

Similarly, the service model also consists of three major types that are listed below:

(a) IaaS (Infrastructure as a Service)
(b) PaaS (Platform as a Service)
(c) SaaS (Software as a Service)

Fig. 15.2 Cloud computing model

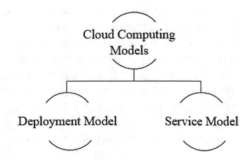

The models and their different types have been explained in detail below. Talking about the deployment model in short, well the deployment model is basically used for the identification part of the cloud environment. This can be based on the basis of the ownership, scalability, the nature of the cloud, the purpose and last but not the least the most significant factor i.e., the accessibility. It is also used to visualize how the infrastructure is going to look like. On the other hand, the Service model lists out the different ways/medium through which the service is provided to the customer/end-user [6] (Fig. 15.3).

It basically gives the end-users/organization a flexible option to choose what kind of service is best for them and then go for the same. Although there are three major types of service models that are listed above but there are also some other service models namely APIaaS, DBaaS etc., and many more that you can choose from. In the next part we will deep dive into the deployment model of Cloud Computing.

Cloud Computing has various applications in many industries like education, finance, real estate, entertainment etc., but due to the outbreak of the Covid-19 pandemic the cloud market has boomed in the healthcare sector as well. If we look at the statistics then as predicted the cloud computing market will be hitting 35 billion dollars by the end of 2022, which is quite a growth. This research was done by BBC [7], which also predicted that the growth rate will be around 12%. Another astonishing fact about cloud computing is that almost 85% of the healthcare sector has switched to the cloud computing. These numbers are self-explanatory that cloud computing has got a lot of applications when it comes to the healthcare sector. Covid-19 has turned out to be one of the biggest threats not only to the human beings but also to many industries like the entertainment industry, transportation

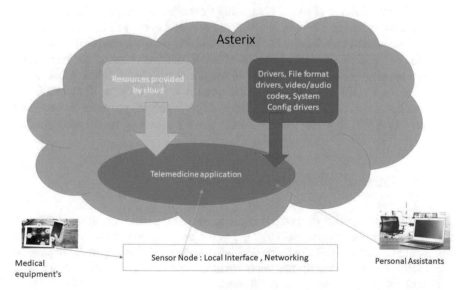

Fig. 15.3 Framework of the secured cloud technology

industry etc. but the only industry that has survived and rise during this time is the healthcare industry. But how did this happen? This happened only because most of the healthcare sector companies have switched to cloud computing and hence, they could easily operate amidst these pandemic times. Various applications of cloud computing include efficient data storage, scalability and the most important aspect i.e., the backing up of the data. Also, since physical interaction wasn't possible amidst these times therefore the patients had to interact using internet which was possible due to cloud computing. Due to the sudden outbreak of the Covid-19 virus the amount of the patient data exploded, had there been no cloud then it would've been very hard to store and manage such a large amount of data. Most of the hospitals switched to video consulting these times which in turn lead to the rise of cloud computing market. Also, the hospitals, that were not using the cloud computing models started to switch to the cloud computing model due to these applications and advantages that it comes up with. Tech Giants like Oracle and IBM also developed cloud architectures amidst these times in order to promote AI research which is cloud based. Cloud also made it possible for the scientists to do research (testing various vaccines) using the data centres that are cloud based. Quick deployment and cost effectiveness are also some additional factors that adds up to the advantages of cloud computing.

Based on the advantages mentioned above there are many applications of Cloud Computing in smart healthcare out of which some are mentioned below:

15.2.2   Medical Records Centralization

Before the introduction of cloud computing in healthcare industry, the data of the patients were stored in multiple handwritten files and every patient had their own separate file which made it quite hard for the hospital staff to manage such data. But since the arrival of the cloud each and every bit of data is now stored at a centralized location which can easily be accessed through a website/web portal. Most of the organisations use AWS S3, or Blob from Azure in order to do so. This data is not only store but also backed up with the help of functionalities provided by the cloud vendors like AWS [8]. Privacy of the data is also taken care of via the same model.

15.2.3   Promoting Patient Engagement

As we all are aware that everything in cloud computing can happen in a matter of few clicks. From increasing data storage to perform any operation everything is a matter of few clicks. Similarly in the healthcare sector with the help of cloud patients can easily schedule their appointments within a few clicks. Also, with the auto reminder facility provide by the AWS notification services namely SMS & Email. Proper monitoring of the data can be done with the help of the cloud computing.

15.2.4   Better Scalability

One of the most significant applications of cloud especially in the healthcare sector is that it is scalable. Now what does Scalability mean? Well Scalability basically means to increase/decrease the data storage space based on the needs of the endusers/organization. Amidst these times of the Covid-19 the amount of patient data gradually increased, but with the scalability that cloud comes up with there was no issue to manage such a huge amount of data. Also cloud vendors like AWS provide functionalities like load balancing and auto scaling which are used by most of the hospitals these days.

15.2.5   Cost-Effectiveness

Another significant of cloud computing is that it is very cost-effective, as mentioned in the earlier part of the document that with cloud you don't need to buy a place, then buy servers and then finally use them. What you can simply do is that you can rent out servers as long as you need also you can scale them according to your needs. Depending on your model that you have chosen; it becomes the responsibility of the cloud vendors to update what is essential. There are various cloud vendors out there like AWS, GCP and Azure that you provide with easy and cost-effective renting and many other cloud based functionalities to choose from [9].

15.2.6   Advanced Analytics for Healthcare

As we all are aware that analytics has the most major role when it comes not to only to the healthcare sector but also in any other sectors. Cloud computing comes to rescue here also, as it provides the data which is stored in the cloud to various machine learning models with the help of which analysis can be done. This model in turn further helps us to visualize and analyse the data effectively. Various cloud vendors provide you the functionality to do such kind of analytics. One of the best examples for the same is the AWS CloudWatch with the help of which helps in the monitoring of the Rest APIs and other content of the website which in turn is quite useful for checking any changes which are unauthorized. These are some of the applications of Cloud Computing in Smart Healthcare. Although there are many more applications but the major ones are mentioned above. Estimated market for cloud at the end of the year 2023 is around 45 billion dollars which is only possible due to the various advantages/applications of the cloud that are mentioned above [10, 11].

15.3   Current and Future Application of AI, IoT, Blockchain and Cloud Computing in Smart Healthcare

15.3.1   Applications of Artificial Intelligence in Smart Healthcare

The application of artificial intelligence and associated technologies in healthcare is just starting. At crucial activities in healthcare, AI has already been shown to perform at least as well as humans. There are many different technologies that make up artificial intelligence (AI).

15.3.2   Machine Learning Neural Networks and Deep Learning

- Computer algorithms mimic intelligent human behaviour and get better with practise.
- This is the main type of artificial intelligence needed for precision medicine.
- A complicated machine learning technique called a neural network is used to predict whether a patient will contract a specific disease by weighing inputs, outputs, and factors or traits that link the three.
- In contrast, deep learning uses a neural network with numerous levels of variables to anticipate results.
- Deep learning is used to identify clinically important aspects in radiological images, where computers are already more accurate than radiologists at identifying cancer occurrences.

15.3.3   Physical Robots

- Robots that can actually move have been used in industry and are therefore widely established.
- Because of advances in AI, they are getting more "intelligent."
- They carry out activities like lifting and welding.
- In the medical context, they distribute supplies.
- Incision-making, wound-sewing, and surgical procedures for head and neck, prostate, and gynecologic surgery can all be done by surgical robots.

15.3.4 Natural Language Processing (NLP)

- NLP focuses on understanding human language and includes tools like speech recognition, text analysis, and objectives.
- The two fundamental NLP methods are statistical and semantic.
- Machine learning is the foundation of statistical natural language processing, and deep learning approaches in particular have improved recognition accuracy.
- NLP systems can examine clinical notes and reports, provide transcription, and create classification schemes for clinical information in the healthcare context.

15.3.5 Applications of Internet of Things (IoT) in Smart Healthcare

A "system of wireless, interconnected, and networked digital devices that can gather, send, and store data via a network without requiring human-to-human or human-to-computer interaction" is what is referred to as the Internet of Things (IoT). IoT can be used in the healthcare industry to refer to any portable device that can assess patient health data and is internet-connected, including computers, smartphones, smart bands and wearables, digital pharmaceuticals, implantable surgical devices, and any other type of portable device. To decide whether it is acceptable to use the IoT to evaluate consumers' and clinicians' degrees of digital literacy, more research is required. Nevertheless, it is believed that the Internet of Things would simplify the delivery of healthcare, from diagnosis to treatment to monitoring of patients inside and outside of the hospital setting.

15.3.6 Applications of Blockchain in Smart Healthcare

- Tracking/registry: The process of transparently and irrevocably storing information and data such that no party has asymmetric control over the information.
- Data access and transfer: Facilitating the sharing of data among several parties to establish a single source of "truth"
- Managing identities and authorizations for authentication or verification, including the capacity to confirm identity characteristics without disclosing sensitive data
- Settlements: Settlement of income via tracking the movement of products and revenues or the use of services and assets
- enabling payments and transactions in (real-time)
- Token exchange: Trading between different parties of virtual money or tokens with intrinsic value. Virtual currencies may also be tied to fiat currencies, with escrow accounts holding the equal value.

15.3.7 Applications of Cloud Computing in Smart Healthcare

E-health and Telemedicine
Nowadays, cloud computing is frequently utilised for e-health, which is the practise of delivering medical services online. Through telesurgery, teleradiology, and other difficult medical issues, the cloud enables collaboration between many medical specialists. Patients living anywhere in the world can receive the appropriate clinical care thanks to e-health. For improved doctor-to-doctor and doctor-to-patient communication and interaction, telemedicine projects leverage cloud computing as an information and communications technology (ICT) infrastructure.

Additionally, cloud-based telemedicine and healthcare applications assist with:

- Sharing patients' medical data in real-time across different geographical locations.
- Minimizing unnecessary visits to hospitals, thereby saving time and money.

Drug Discovery
Drug recovery necessitates a substantial amount of processing power to find unique molecules among billions of chemical structures, hence cloud computing is crucial in this process. Services that provide infrastructure as a service (IaaS) are particularly helpful in streamlining this procedure.

Healthcare Information Systems
Cloud-based management information systems are used by the healthcare sector to improve patient care, administer human resources, better query services, and handle invoicing and finances. Development, testing, and deployment of these systems are all done using cloud computing in the healthcare sector. Cloud computing facilitates cross-platform interoperability, quick, collaborative development, and greater system integration with other healthcare systems.

15.4 Challenges in Smart Healthcare

Although Cloud Computing comes up with various advantages and applications that are mentioned above which includes some of the key advantages like cost-effectiveness, scalability, analytics etc. but there are still some areas especially when in it comes to healthcare sector where cloud computing faces certain challenges which must be overcome in future in order to make Cloud Computing even more powerful in the healthcare sector. One of the most interesting facts to notice here while looking at the challenges of the cloud computing is that certain advantages that cloud offers often leads to the disadvantages/challenges. One such factor here is the centralization of data, now we all know that how useful centralization of data is, especially in healthcare sector as it acts as a one place solution for the staff to access and retrieve those records easily, but another thing here to notice is that it also leads to rise of the security and the privacy related concerns. Even for the attackers also the centralized data acts as a one stop solution and they can retrieve that data and use it to their needs which in turn is not good. There are many other areas like these where cloud computing needs to be improved and solutions must be provided in these areas to tackle these privacy related concerns. Cloud Computing, especially the public cloud is open and anyone can access it according to their needs, this also leads to one of the major privacy and security related concerns. Hackers/Attackers can steal, modify data which can lead to wrong analysis and can lead to the downfall of the organisation. This is one of the most severe problems which needs to be fixed as quickly as possible. This is one the major reasons why some of the healthcare organizations are still hesitating to switch over to cloud. As we all are aware that the cloud vendors can store data in multiple data centres that can be present at different geographical locations which can be useful when it comes to the data backup but the same advantage can lead to one of the biggest disadvantages i.e., data theft. This can be explained very easily as the data is present at different data centres which are in turn located in different locations this can increase the chances of the data theft. Another major challenge that the cloud computing model is facing in healthcare is the improper encryption. There are certain parameters that the cloud computing models/cloud vendors should meet, these include keeping the records of the patients confidential, making sure that the integrity of the data is maintained and the data that is being stored is accurate, the data should be available within few clicks and the staff/end-user should not be kept waiting for a large interval of time to retrieve the data that they want. Adding up, the data that is being stored should be authentic and no modifications should be done that hampers it authenticity, there should the features to capture and verify the digital signatures as soon as anyone updates a certain record so that if any unforeseen circumstances arise in the future, then one can always trace back to the person who last modified the records. A proper encryption mechanism should be provided by the cloud vendors so that the patient remains anonymous and the hackers/attackers can't steal the records on the basis of a certain patient. Last but not the least these functionalities should be properly maintained by the cloud vendors.

Above mentioned are some of the points that should be met the cloud vendors which are providing the cloud computing services. Now we are going to look in brief about the challenges that cloud faces in the healthcare sector. These are as follows:

15.4.1 Availability

One of the major limitations when it comes to cloud computing is that the service that is provided by the cloud vendors can sometimes be slow. Almost everyone of us at some point of time must have heard that the server went down, this is what can happen with cloud computing. Also, as we all know that cloud heavily relies on the network connection, so if the internet connection is not good then it lead to a bad user experience which can turn out to be one of the major limitations.

15.4.2   Data Centralization

As mentioned above that data centralization which is one of the major advantages of cloud computing is also one of the biggest limitations of cloud computing. It leads to rise of the security and the privacy related concerns as the hackers/attackers might easily steal and tamper the data in case of absence of proper cloud security. They can retrieve that data and use it to their needs which in turn is not safe for the privacy of the patients.

15.4.3   Privacy/Security

Data privacy/security is one of the major limitations when it comes to cloud. As we all are aware that the cloud vendors can store data in multiple data centres that can be present at different geographical locations which can be useful when it comes to the data backup but the same advantage can lead to one of the biggest disadvantages i.e., data theft. As the data is present at different data centres which are in turn located in different locations this can increase the chances of the data theft.

15.4.4   Open Access

Last but not the least open access which is also one of the advantages of cloud computing is also another limitation of cloud computing. Since, the public cloud is open and anyone can access it according to their needs, this also leads to one of the major privacy and security related concerns. Hackers/Attackers can steal, modify data which can lead to wrong analysis and can lead to the downfall of the organisation.

These were some of the major limitations of cloud computing which needs to be tackled so that cloud computing can become reliable in the field of healthcare. Although cloud computing has got multiple applications but there are some areas where it needs to improve to make it more efficient in the field of healthcare.

15.5   Future of Smart Healthcare and Telemedicine

With 76% of purchasers expressing interest in the use of telehealth in the destiny, and the capability of telehealth to resolve longstanding challenges in healthcare delivery, companies have a vested interest in finding ways to integrate telehealth into their care fashions. However, growing long-time period telehealth strategies will require cautious assessment of foundational technology. For instance, businesses are exploring structures that offer integrated communications, robust security, scalability for surge demand, and far way control abilities. During a webinar, Gregg Malkary, Founder and Managing Director of Spyglass Consulting, presented new research from a white paper developed in partnership with Ring Central surveying healthcare providers that correctly deployed telehealth. This studies examines the critical considerations companies must explore while choosing telehealth answers and highlights the capability of the cloud. Successfully deployed telehealth Solutions can direct patient-focused care models that may maximise value-based compensation and that can help achieve the Quadruple framework by lowering health care costs, enhancing care quality and outcomes, and promoting affected person outreach and engagement, according to Malkary.

A cloud telemedicine is a solution with some specifications they are:

- Integrated communication: Devices that can transmit relaxed, high-fidelity audio and video for both scheduled and on-demand appointments, in addition to comfortable text-based communications, as well as integrations that permit the sharing of digital clinical imaging and patient fitness statistics.
- Diverse cellular endpoints: Allow for communication with hospitals and carriers using exceptional computing devices. Platforms should also enable patient communication via their preferred device, whether it be a computer, tablet, mobile phone, or landline.
- The use of middleware to ensure seamless integration with administrative procedures, such as scheduling, and EHRs [12, 13].
- Centralized management, including exact use reviews, to improve medical workflow processes, address networking problems, and demonstrate the return on investment of telehealth packages.
- Enterprise-level security, such as gold-level HITRUST certification, to meet HIP compliance regulations and protect sensitive patient statistics. This should include host controls, password-protected meetings, and encrypted statistics transfer to assist identify and validate assembly attendees (Fig. 15.4).

According to an old proverb, need is the mother of invention. The immediate need to provide nutritional options during COVID-19 has shown the potential and specifications for gold-standard care delivery via telehealth. By employing continuity of care presentations, telehealth played a key role in establishing connections between clinicians and patients during COVID-19. It saved patient lives, decreased the risk of viral transmission, allowed doctors to spend more time with patients, and increased access to care, particularly for patients who may reside in underserved urban and rural areas, according to Malkary. And since telehealth is here to stay, health care corporations must provide the 24/7 access to care that today's patients want. Implementing cloud-based, fully telehealth-based next-generation health care technologies should be a core component of each enterprise's virtual health strategy.

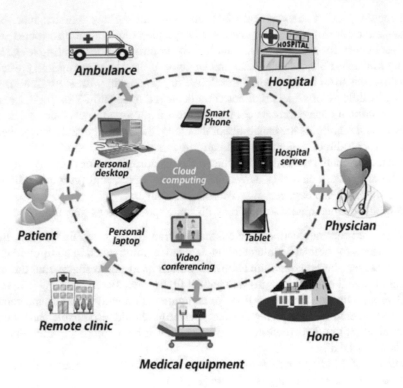

Fig. 15.4 Future of telemedicine

15.6 Conclusion

The Telemedicine system will face quite a lot of problems in the present because both the doctor and the patient won't be familiar with its working. It'll take a lot of time for everyone to properly understand how it works, if one of the parties involved doesn't knows how the system works it will cause a communication gap. There would be a lot of security breaches in the start because its hard to maintain the network and share the data between them in a moment. Telemedicine system will cost quite a bit because the cloud storage doesn't come for free nor the staff to maintain such a huge system. But in the distant future telemedicine system will become the best thing that humanity would've invested in terms of health. With time the AI will progress and will be so good that it could suggest prescription to the patient based on his health problems. The IoT devices would grow at a fast pace and would be advanced enough to give a very precise health record as well as would be able to measure other health stats. Blockchain would enhance the security and immediate response to the next level. Hopefully the cost of this system will be affordable for the common mass because cloud computing would become more versatile and enhanced. In conclusion, in the future because of the advancement of each IT sector the technologies would be so enhanced that it'll be a wise decision to spend time and labour to create this type of system to take a step to a healthy lifestyle.

References

1. Huang, G.-B., Zhu, Q.-Y. & Siew, C.-K. Extreme learning machine: Theory and applications. Neurocomputing 70, 489–501 (2006).
2. Hitesh Kumar Sharma; Anuj Kumar; Sangeeta Pant; Mangey Ram, "8 Electronic Healthcare Record (EHR) Storage using Blockchain for Smart Healthcare," in Artificial Intelligence, Blockchain and IoT for Smart Healthcare, River Publishers, 2022, pp. 77–84.
3. Hitesh Kumar Sharma; Anuj Kumar; Sangeeta Pant; Mangey Ram, "9 Methodologies for Improving the Quality of Service and Safety of Smart Healthcare," in Artificial Intelligence, Blockchain and IoT for Smart Healthcare, River Publishers, 2022, pp. 85–94.
4. Hitesh Kumar Sharma; Anuj Kumar; Sangeeta Pant; Mangey Ram, "10 Cloud Commuting Platform for Smart Healthcare and Telemedicine," in Artificial Intelligence, Blockchain and IoT for Smart Healthcare, River Publishers, 2022, pp. 95–104.
5. Nguyen, G. et al. ML and DL frameworks and libraries for substantial and ample data mining: A survey. Artif. Intell. Rev. 52, 77–124 (2019).
6. Kshitiz, K., et al. "Detecting hate speech and insults on social commentary using NLP and machine learning." International Journal of Engineering Technology Science and Research 4.12 (2017): 279–285.
7. Hitesh Kumar Sharma; Anuj Kumar; Sangeeta Pant; Mangey Ram, "4 Application of Artificial Intelligence in Smart Healthcare," in Artificial Intelligence, Blockchain and IoT for Smart Healthcare, River Publishers, 2022, pp. 37–46.
8. Hitesh Kumar Sharma; Anuj Kumar; Sangeeta Pant; Mangey Ram, "5 Application of IoT in Smart Healthcare," in Artificial Intelligence, Blockchain and IoT for Smart Healthcare, River Publishers, 2022, pp. 47–56.
9. Hitesh Kumar Sharma; Anuj Kumar; Sangeeta Pant; Mangey Ram, "6 Application of Blockchain in Smart Healthcare," in Artificial Intelligence, Blockchain and IoT for Smart Healthcare, River Publishers, 2022, pp. 57–66.
10. Hitesh Kumar Sharma; Anuj Kumar; Sangeeta Pant; Mangey Ram, "7 Security and Privacy challenge in Smart Healthcare and Telemedicine systems," in Artificial Intelligence, Blockchain and IoT for Smart Healthcare, River Publishers, 2022, pp. 67–76.
11. Hitesh Kumar Sharma; Anuj Kumar; Sangeeta Pant; Mangey Ram, "8 Electronic Healthcare Record (EHR) Storage using Blockchain for Smart Healthcare," in Artificial Intelligence, Blockchain and IoT for Smart Healthcare, River Publishers, 2022, pp. 77–84.
12. Hitesh Kumar Sharma; Anuj Kumar; Sangeeta Pant; Mangey Ram, "9 Methodologies for Improving the Quality of Service and Safety of Smart Healthcare," in Artificial Intelligence, Blockchain and IoT for Smart Healthcare, River Publishers, 2022, pp. 85–94.
13. Hitesh Kumar Sharma; Anuj Kumar; Sangeeta Pant; Mangey Ram, "10 Cloud Commuting Platform for Smart Healthcare and Telemedicine," in Artificial Intelligence, Blockchain and IoT for Smart Healthcare, River Publishers, 2022, pp. 95–104.